Nubia Katia Teixeira

The operation of a converted traditional health centre

Nubia Katia Teixeira

The operation of a converted traditional health centre

Family Health Strategy

ScienciaScripts

Imprint

Any brand names and product names mentioned in this book are subject to trademark, brand or patent protection and are trademarks or registered trademarks of their respective holders. The use of brand names, product names, common names, trade names, product descriptions etc. even without a particular marking in this work is in no way to be construed to mean that such names may be regarded as unrestricted in respect of trademark and brand protection legislation and could thus be used by anyone.

Cover image: www.ingimage.com

This book is a translation from the original published under ISBN 978-613-9-73197-8.

Publisher:
Sciencia Scripts
is a trademark of
Dodo Books Indian Ocean Ltd. and OmniScriptum S.R.L publishing group

120 High Road, East Finchley, London, N2 9ED, United Kingdom
Str. Armeneasca 28/1, office 1, Chisinau MD-2012, Republic of Moldova, Europe
Printed at: see last page
ISBN: 978-620-7-88913-6

SUMMARY

Introduction: The Family Health Strategy emerged in the context of public health to reorient the care service and strengthen the basic principles of the SUS, with the aim of replacing or converting the traditional model of primary care. In 2006, the process of converting Health Centre 03 in Samambaia - DF began, and there was a need to evaluate its functioning after the conversion. **General objective:** To assess the relationship between the existing organisational structure and that recommended for a Health Centre converted to the Family Health Strategy. **Specific objectives: To** analyse the perception of the professionals in the family health team about the way the unit works; to compare the perception of the professionals with the reality observed by the researchers; to assess whether the organisation of the work process in the converted health unit is in line with what is recommended by the Ministry of Health, reporting any points of disagreement. **Methodology:** This is a descriptive observational qualitative study carried out at the 03 Samambaia Health Centre between April 2009 and April 2010, with data collection divided into two parts: a semi-structured interview and a participant observation study. The interviews were analysed using Bardin's method. Ordinance 648/2006 was mainly used to assess the functioning of the centre. The observation was described as it was followed during the established period and a comparative table was drawn up. **Discussion: There** was evidence of greater involvement between the professionals and the population, a broadening of the forms of **professional** action **and an improvement in resolutiveness. The conversion process was "traumatic" for the** staff and the lack of prior training accentuated this difficulty. The profile of the manager, their length of stay and standardisations interfere with the smooth running of the strategy, as do the motivation and profile of the professionals working in it. Demand was found to be twice as high as that recommended by decree 648/2006 and complaints of insufficient physical space. Teamwork, which was highly emphasised as a positive point, allows for joint planning and specific strategies for each catchment area. On the other hand, continuing education only takes place at central level, leaving no time for in-house training, which is carried out on an ad hoc basis. The observation found a great deal of agreement between the activities recommended and those carried out, but the high demand and bureaucratic activities hinder home visits by the doctor and nurse and the monthly visit by the ACS. **Final considerations:** The initial proposal for the family health programme corresponds to the needs of the community and would be effective if applied with adequate demand and sufficient resources. However, the conversion was only successful due to the commitment and involvement of all the professionals and depends on incentives from all spheres of government. The converted health unit must be seen as a third structure that is more complex than its formative parts and new norms must emerge to structure and evaluate its development. **Recommendations:** There should be prior training for the professionals who will work in the new model; offer enough teams to cover the unit's catchment area; provide adequate physical space, if not inside, in areas adjacent to the unit, appoint a local manager committed to the family health strategy and its operation; involve all the managers of the strategy, at regional and central level, with the whole process.

Key words: Family Health, conversion, primary care.

Summary

CHAPTER 1

INTRODUCTION

The Family Health Strategy (Estratégia Saúde da Família - ESF) emerged in Brazil as a new plan to reorient the care model based on primary care, in line with the principles of the Unified Health System (Sistema Único de Saúde - SUS), bringing new perspectives to health care for the population, and advocated to be the main gateway to the service network. In addition, the practice of family health care is seen as integral, humanised and takes into account an equitable approach through clinical and territorial responsibility.

The Ministry of Health supported this initiative by changing the name of Family Health, which was created as a programme, and now it is considered by the Ministry of Health itself to be a structuring strategy for municipal health systems, aimed at reorienting the care model and creating a new dynamic in the organisation of health services and actions. [27]

The aim of this strategy is to replace or convert the traditional model of health care, historically characterised as attending to spontaneous demand, eminently curative, hospital-centred, high-cost, without establishing hierarchical networks by complexity, with low resolutiveness and in which the health team does not establish bonds of cooperation and co-responsibility with the community.

In the traditional model, health posts or centres worked without commitment to the community and were often limited to vaccinating children, attending outpatient appointments and constantly referring patients to hospitals. Today, the Family Health Units work within a new logic, with greater capacity to respond to the population's basic health needs. [3]

In order for primary care to be of high quality, it is necessary to have professionals who are responsible and committed to the community to work in this strategy. [11]

The Family Health model is a strategy for organising primary health care that can be presented under the following conceptions: a) a strategy for reordering the health sector, which means affecting and understanding the entire health system and the entire population that this system is supposed to serve; b) a programme with restricted objectives, specifically designed to satisfy some elementary and predetermined needs of human groups considered to be in a situation of extreme poverty and marginalisation, with differentiated resources, low technological density and minimal costs; and c) a strategy for organising the first level of care in the health system. [8]

The formulation of the Family Health Strategy incorporated the basic principles of the SUS - universalisation, decentralisation, comprehensiveness and community participation - and was developed on the basis of the Family Health Team (ESF), which works by defining a catchment area, enrolling clients, registering and monitoring the population of the area, which should be up to a maximum of 4,000 people, with an average of 3,000 people recommended for each team. [4]

The Family Health Team is multi-professional, consisting of at least a general practitioner, a nurse, a nursing assistant and four to six Community Health Agents (ACS). Within the National Primary Care Policy, each professional has common and specific duties. [4]

As already mentioned, the Family Health Unit (USF) is considered the gateway and the first level of care, and must be integrated into a network of services at different levels of complexity, establishing a system of referrals and counter-referrals that guarantee resolution and enable patients to be monitored. [2]

On the basis of the Ministry of Health's proposal, with the initiative of the Director of Primary Care and Family Health Strategy (DIAPS) and with the full support of the then director of the Samambaia Regional Health Department in 2006, an important step was taken in an attempt to reorganise primary care in the Federal District, which was the conversion of Samambaia Health Centre No. 3. This is a satellite city of the Federal District, with around 170,000 inhabitants, according to the IBGE, but this is an underestimated population, as according to a survey by the Samambaia Regional Administration, the city already has over 200,000 inhabitants. Like all satellite towns, it is financially dependent on the Federal District government, but it has a good urban infrastructure with 100 per cent water supply from CAESB, and around 95 per cent tarmac and sewage, as well as public rubbish collection throughout the city. In addition, local commerce is growing every day with the emergence of various liberal activities such as clinics, as well as a promising property and construction market.

Samambaia has a small health network in view of its population, made up of just four Health Centres and a medium-sized Regional Hospital, as well as a private hospital and some small clinics. The Health Centre that is the setting for this research has its own characteristics, such as a population, according to the IBGE, of just over 13,640 inhabitants, located in a distinct geographical area, around 1 km away from the rest of the city. It was precisely because of this peculiarity that DIAPS chose it as the place to carry out the conversion.

The importance of this work arises from the need to assess the functioning of the health unit after the conversion process, since there is doubt among the professionals who work there as to whether the functioning of the unit is as recommended by the Ministry of Health. This doubt persists due to the great difficulty in looking for models similar to the one sought in other places to follow as an example.

This work could serve as a source of research for other basic health units that are converted from the traditional model to the family health strategy.

In view of the above, the general objective of this research project is to evaluate the organisational structure of a traditional health centre converted into a Family Health Strategy, in accordance with the recommendations of the Ministry of Health.

At the end of this study, we hope to get to know the real situation of the health unit in question, in terms of how it works and how it is organised, given that it was a health centre that was converted in its entirety to the family health strategy. In addition, it is necessary to propose improvements and, to this end, knowing exactly where interventions are needed would help in the process of overcoming the existing organisation and achieving what everyone wants.

CHAPTER 2

Objectives

2.1.   General Objective

To assess the relationship between the existing organisational structure and the recommended structure of a Health Centre converted into a Family Health Strategy.

2.2.   Specific objectives

- To analyse the perception of family health team professionals about the functioning of the unit.
- To compare the professional's perception with the reality observed by the researchers.
- Evaluate whether the organisation of the health unit's work process is in line with what is recommended by the Ministry of Health, reporting any points of disagreement.

CHAPTER 3

Methodology

The research problem in question aims to answer a constant doubt among the staff at Samambaia's Health Centre No. 03 about its operation, which is whether the conversion has been completed in accordance with what the Ministry of Health recommends. There is a lot of talk among staff about the differences that exist between the way the unit works and what the Ministry of Health describes in its regulations on the Family Health Strategy, especially in Ministerial Order MS 648/2006.

In order to answer this problem, it was initially planned to use the Quality Improvement Assessment (QIA), available from the Ministry of Health, to assess the Family Health Strategy. However, when the document in question was read, it was concluded that the conversion had been completed recently, with various events and management and organisational complications at the SHS-DF that would prevent the QIA from being applied reliably in the Health Unit that is the subject of this research. [25]

In view of this, it was decided to evaluate the functioning of the converted health unit by comparing what is recommended by the Ministry of Health with what was done in the Samambaia Health Centre No. 03, through Ordinance 648/2006, and also through the perception of the health professionals who work in the unit in question.

This project is a descriptive observational qualitative study, with data collection consisting of two stages, the first of which was a semi-structured interview with the staff of the Samambaia Health Centre No. 03. As an inclusion criterion, we chose to interview all the staff who were registered with the three Family Health teams, which comprise: three doctors, three nurses, ten nursing technicians and nine community health agents. In addition, the questionnaire was also administered to the heads of the health unit, which include the Health Centre Manager; the Head of Nursing; the Head of Administration; and the Head of the Regulation, Control and Assessment Centre (NRCA). The same questions applied to the other professionals could be used to enrich the conversion assessment. It was decided not to include support professionals as administrative staff, due to the lack of parameters to compare with what is recommended by the Ministry of Health, as well as excluding staff from the NASF, which exists in the unit, since it was set up two years after the conversion and deserves to be the subject of a specific study.

The second stage was a participant observation study, in which the researchers were involved in the team's daily work in order to extract the full reality of the situation.

The data collection technique is guided by the best method, according to the researcher's objectives. In the case of this research, the two techniques chosen are justified so that one complements the data collected through the other, with the aim of producing versions of the world, without losing the notion that knowledge is always a construction of the collective, in other words, a construction of reality. [14]

Bardin's content analysis was used to analyse the results of the interview. Its aim is to analyse the characteristics of a message by comparing these messages for different recipients, or in different situations with the same recipients. To this end, analytical reading is used as an instrument to carry out the analysis, which is also classified as categorical, according to Bardin's definition, and the so-called pre-analysis must first be carried out, consisting of textual and thematic analysis and the analysis itself. [20]

Next, the elements must be categorised (**a *priori or a posteriori*) *in*** order to analyse and process the information. This phase is followed by the substantive exploration of the material and, finally, the treatment of the results, inference and interpretation. [20]

Qualitative research works with many meanings, motivations, aspirations, beliefs, values and attitudes, which leads to a deeper understanding of relationships, processes and phenomena. The researcher is an active discoverer of the meaning of actions and relationships that are hidden in social structures. [21,14]

Therefore, with qualitative research we can draw out the most intimate aspects of it, since in the case of the project in question we are working with people in their workplace, which leads to the collection of various meanings for the object of the research. It is essential to comment on the care taken in collecting and analysing the data, precisely because of the amount of information that was collected and transposed. [14]

In view of this need for care, the researchers were trained in the qualitative approach and in the data collection techniques chosen for this research before these stages began. They were also trained in the data analysis chosen, Bardin's content analysis, which was crucial for the proper development of the work. However, not all the students in the group were able to take part, as we only had two students for a while due to the withdrawal of two others, and only after about three months were two more students included in the work. The only damage caused by this was the delay in data collection, but we guided these new students in both collecting and analysing the data and the commitment of the old students to teaching the new ones, and of the latter to learning, meant that the development of this research did not suffer any major damage.

The semi-structured interview used in the first stage allowed the interviewer greater flexibility, in that they could change the order of the questions and had ample freedom to make interventions according to the progress of the interview. [14]

This type of interview is widely used when you want to limit the volume of information, thus obtaining a greater focus on the topic, intervening so that the objectives are achieved. [22]

Precisely because of these possibilities, the questions in the semi-structured interview, which are open-ended, underwent minor modifications, according to the needs assessed during the process of getting to know the Health Unit, the setting for this research.

This was an individual interview, to preserve the integrity of the answers, with four questions: **"What is your role within this unit?"; "What** changes have you observed in the functioning of CSSam 03 with the conversion?"; **"What positive points** would you highlight as most relevant in the functioning of Health Centre No. 03 in **Samambaia? (Name three)"; "What negative points would you highlight as most relevant in**

the functioning of Health Centre No. 03 in Samambaia? (Name three)".

In the second stage of the research, data will be collected through participant observation, taking into account that to observe is to apply the senses in order to obtain certain information about some aspect of reality. It is through the intellectual act of observing the phenomenon under study that a real notion of the being or natural environment is conceived, as a direct source of data. [23]

Participant observation is aimed at describing the components of a situation in great detail, experiencing and understanding the dynamics of acts and events and collecting data based on the understanding and meaning that the actors attribute to their own actions. This form of data collection fulfils the objectives of this research, as it complements the information collected through interviews. [24,23]

The researchers stayed for two months, on non-consecutive days that were defined according to their availability, with a weekly presence of 4 hours at the unit, observing the functioning of all the activities of the three teams at the Health Centre, and taking notes of all the information in the various sectors of the unit. This period was important in order to be able to follow all the team's daily activities, which are different for each professional category, and consist of home visits by all the professionals, consultations for prenatal care, child growth and development (CD), paediatrics, gynaecology and clinical medicine, carried out by the doctor; nursing consultations, prenatal care, CD, colpocytology consultations, carried out by the nurse; educational meetings, held by the doctor, nurse and nursing technicians, as well as nursing procedures generally carried out by the technicians, and various activities carried out by the CHAs. The researchers were then inserted into the context of each team and wrote down all the information in a pre-established script, which is attached.

The first stage was pre-analysis, based on a floating reading of the transcripts and notes taken by the interviewers. This was done in pairs, where each person read the other's interviews several times in order to grasp the content and extract themes that could be grouped into categories.

In a second stage, the themes were grouped into the following categories:
1. Staff perception of the improvement in patient care with the converted model;
2. Teamwork in the development of care actions;
3. Influence of personal motivation on the functioning of the Centre and personal opinions on the ESF;
4. Reflections on the conversion process;
5. The relationship between physical structure, staff and demand on the quality of care;
6. Continuing education;
7. Influence of existing standardisation and management on strategy performance.

To finalise the analysis, it was processed and described according to the categories found in the results of this research. The data was then analysed against the Ministry of Health's current regulatory documents.

In this way, it was possible to come to a conclusion about how Samambaia's Health Centre No. 03 is working, and whether it is possible to follow the Ministry of Health's recommendations with the conversion.

CHAPTER 4

Contextualising the research problem

4.1. Conceptualisation

The Family Health Programme (PSF) was officially created in 1994 as a strategy by the Ministry of Health to reorganise the municipal health system. This means that it can replace the old guidelines focussing on hospital and curative care for illness and introduce new principles focussing on health promotion and community participation. [2]

The Ministry of Health defines the Family Health Programme as the gateway to the health system, which must be regionalised and hierarchical. In addition, as explained above, it is necessary to define an area of activity with a well-defined population that is the team's responsibility. [1]

The family and the environment in which it lives is the main focus of the strategy, and as functions the PSF has to provide comprehensive, permanent and quality care, carry out health education and promotion activities, bring the community to participate in the actions of the health unit, make use of health information systems for monitoring and decision-making, act in epidemiological surveillance, work with prevention, but not forgetting health recovery, assisting the patient at home whenever necessary. [11]

In his study on family health, Goulart (2002) cites SOUSA (2001), who defines the PSF with certain characteristics, such as health as a right of access to goods and services, not just assistance; health promotion; health for all and primary health care; community action for health; advocacy in favour of health; healthy environments and support for health; social involvement; self-help; sustainable development, as well as the proposal for healthy cities. [1]

The Family Health model is a strategy for organising primary health care that can be presented in the following terms: a) a strategy for reorganising the health sector, which means affecting and understanding the entire health system and the entire population that this system is supposed to serve; b) a programme with restricted objectives, specifically designed to meet certain elementary and predetermined needs of human groups considered to be in a situation of extreme poverty and marginalisation, with differentiated resources, low technological density and minimal costs; and c) a strategy for organising the first level of care in the health system. [8]

The PSF can guarantee the quality, comprehensiveness and effectiveness of the first level of care, or it can aim for technologically simplified care for the low-income population. In addition, the programme is capable of selective action to reduce costs. [9]

Responding to criticisms that Family Health is, in reality, a "SUS for the poor", with low resolubility and verticalisation, the Ministry of Health highlights the transformative potential of the proposal, whose guidelines are consistent with the fundamental principles of the system. Although labelled as a programme, the PSF escapes the usual conception of the others, as it is not a vertical intervention, parallel to the activities of the health services. It falls within the scope of the health system, which is made up of a hierarchical and regionalised network; thus, its implementation does not mean the creation of new service structures, except in deprived areas, but rather the replacement of conventional care practices with a new work process, with universal coverage, which exempts it from being characterised as a health system aimed at low-income people.[10]

In light of the above, the conversion of Health Centre No. 03 in Samambaia has been in line with the replacement proposed by the Ministry of Health, further emphasising the need to evaluate this replacement in order to find out how the changes have taken place and their impact on the work of the professionals who work in this unit.

The Family Health Programme is currently being defended by the Ministry of Health as a strategy for reorienting the healthcare model. According to Testa,[7] the concept of **Strategy** refers to the way in which a policy is implemented; in this sense, it constitutes **"organisational behaviour aimed at managing situations in which it is necessary to overcome obstacles that stand in the way of achieving an objective"**. The term can also be understood as **"a way of realising a policy"**, which ultimately means a given redistribution of power in the health sector and/or in society.[6]

Professionals working in the Family Health Strategy, in their individual and/or collective clinical practice, should always seek to..:[11]

- A holistic approach to the health-disease process;
- Integral, interdisciplinary and intersectoral;
- Strong doctor-patient relationship, producing autonomy;
- Use of scientifically based knowledge and tools;
- Emphasis on health promotion and disease prevention;
- Early diagnosis of problems and diseases;
- Attention to new health problems;
- Continued care for chronic problems; and
- Timely prevention.

The definition of how the family health unit works is better explained in the following sections.

4.2. Territory and population

A family health team is responsible for a specific territory with a population of up to 1,000 families and no more than 4,000 people.[4]

According to the Ministry of Health's parameters, portrayed in Ordinance GM/ MS 648/2006, a health unit in large urban centres should have no more than 3 teams, which generates a population of around 12,000 people. [4]

Defining the territory in which each team will operate is the first step in setting up family health teams. The territory is actually an area where there are people, businesses and institutions that are interrelated and influenced by economic, social, environmental, cultural and political factors.[11]

This area needs to go through the process of territorialisation, which is continuous and serves to identify geographical aspects, such as the presence of hills and rivers that can interfere with access to the health unit; socio-demographic aspects, such as socio-economic profile, presence of institutions, commerce, among others; and epidemiological aspects, such as areas of health risk, presence of water and sewage networks, energy, rubbish collection, vacant lots. It is also important to look at the means of transport in the area. [11]

This territorialisation serves to give an overview of the team's area of operation, and which priorities should be taken into account when starting the team's work. It also serves to make initial contact with the population in order to get to know their customs and habits and to draw up action strategies. [11]

It also serves to divide the area into micro-areas for each community health agent to work in, with each one's population not exceeding 250 families or 750 people. [4]

In order to consolidate territorialisation, a widely used tool is mapping, in which a map of the area is made and everything that has been collected through territorialisation is placed there in symbols and colours.

Finally, registration begins, which consolidates the start of the family health unit's activities for the population. Registration is carried out by the ACS, through a home visit and using the Ficha A - Ficha de Cadastramento Familiar (Family Registration Form), from which information is used for surveillance and planning the team's activities. This form is part of the SIAB (Primary Care Information System) database, used by the Ministry of Health to monitor the strategy in all Brazilian states. [11]

4.3. Human Resources

According to Decree 648/2006, the teams are made up of a minimum of one doctor, one nurse, a nursing assistant and Community Health Workers (CHWs), enough to cover 100 per cent of the team's area, working in units that can have between one and three teams. [3,4]

To this composition can be added an oral health team, which in its modality 1 is made up of a dental surgeon and a dental office assistant, and can be reinforced by the presence of a dental hygiene technician (modality 2). An oral health team can be responsible for a maximum of two family health teams.

The daily workload for all PSF professionals must be 8 hours, totalling 40 hours a week. [4]

The team can include other professionals, depending on the interest of the managers and the needs of the service. It's very common for there to be an administrative assistant who organises files, medical records and also types up the SIAB. In addition, the Ministry of Health recently created the NASF - Family Health Support Centre, which has two types, NASF 1 and 2, depending on which professional categories are present in each. It was created to support specialists who work in primary care, such as gynaecologists, paediatricians, clinicians, physiotherapists, social workers, nutritionists and others. The main aim of the NASF is to provide support to general practitioners and the entire family health team, who often have nowhere to refer problems that can be solved in the primary care network, simply by having the presence of a specialist there.

4.4. Physical structure and supplies

There are no rigid rules for the physical structure of basic units, but they must take into account the four basic elements of PHC, which are first contact access, longitudinality, comprehensiveness and coordination. Spaces should be used in a shared way, remembering that teamwork is a premise of the PSF. [11]

There are physical area specifications in the Ministry of Health's Manual for the Physical Structure of Basic Health Units: Family Health, 2006, which give all the suggestions on how to have an adequate physical structure for one, two or even three family health teams in the same physical space, including the necessary equipment.

According to the Ministry of Health's Ordinance 648/2006, the basic unit needs to be registered in the Ministry of Health's General Register of Health Establishments, and should minimally have: a doctor's and nurse's office for the team, a reception area/room, a place for files and records, a room for basic nursing care, a vaccination room and toilets, as well as adequate equipment and materials for the list of planned actions to ensure that the care provided is effective.

The physical structure must be appropriate to the reality of the situation, with basic equipment that is indispensable for providing good service to the community. [3,4]

It is also necessary to guarantee referral and counter-referral flows to specialised, diagnostic and therapeutic support, outpatient and inpatient services, and there must also be permanent maintenance of the supplies needed to care for the population. [4]

4.5. Permanent education

The training process should begin together with the implementation of the teams, and it is recommended that all team members be trained within 30 days. Municipalities with more than 100,000 inhabitants, such as Brasília, should be responsible for providing training. [4]
After the introductory training, which should be done by all members of the family health team, the process of permanent education begins in the day-to-day running of the unit, which enables the constant development of their competences as a generalist team. [2]

It's important to include a period in the weekly schedule for continuing education for the whole team, which can begin with discussions of clinical cases of patients who have been present in the unit, or whose

CHAs have brought them as an example, and who have questions. From there, a permanent education schedule can be set up with content that covers all the stages of the life cycle, incorporating everyone's experiences of working within the family health strategy into each training session.

The Ministry of Health (2002) suggests the following project:

Child Health Module	Nutritional surveillance, vaccination, care for prevalent childhood diseases
Adolescent Health Module	Actions to promote adolescent health.
Women's Health Module	Prenatal care; cervical cancer prevention and family planning
Adult Health Module	Actions to control diabetes mellitus, hypertension and promote workers' health.
Elderly Health Module	Actions to promote the quality of life and health of the elderly.
Tuberculosis Control	Active search for cases, clinical diagnosis, supervised treatment of BK+ cases, treatment and follow-up of BK- cases, and other actions to prevent and control tuberculosis.
Leprosy elimination	Active search for cases, clinical diagnosis, registration of carriers, supervised treatment of cases, control of physical disabilities and other preventive measures.
Oral Health Module	Clinical care, health promotion and actions to control and stabilise oral pathologies with a view to self-care.

Continuing education also has a number of priorities: violence, drugs, prostitution, children at risk, mental health, oral health, workers' health, STDs/AIDS, social exclusion, citizenship, human rights, social and urban movements.

4.6.   History of the PSF

In an attempt to change the country's health system, Brazil enacted the Unified Health System (SUS) in the 1988 Constitution, which had already been discussed at the 8ª National Health Conference **in 1986. With the creation of the SUS, it was defined that health "is a right of all and a duty of the state", and the organisation of the system must follow certain guidelines, which are:**

> **(...) I- decentralisation, with a single directorate in each sphere of government;**
>
> **II- comprehensive care, with priority given to preventive activities, without prejudice to care services;**
>
> **III- community participation (...)**

However, even before the Constitution was promulgated, some initiatives were already taking place in some places in Brazil, such as the Community Health Agents Programme, which began in 1987 in the state of Ceará.

The Family Health Programme is part of Brazil's recent history, but its primordial ideas date back to the beginning of medicine, when doctors' main activity was their consulting rooms, which were usually set up in their own homes, and care was provided there, in full view of the families or often in the homes of those who came to see them.[1]

Over the centuries, medicine changed and so did the care models, with the 20th century being marked by curative medicine and the explosion of specialities, in parallel with the health campaigns that had been taking place since the beginning of the century. [1]

Attempts to talk about family health or family medicine were made throughout the 1970s and 1980s, but contradictions about the model and resistance to it caused countless discussions in various sectors involved in health, from the Ministry to the Medical Council, political parties and even universities. [1]

4.6.1. The PSF in the world

The positive impact of Primary Health Care (PHC) in achieving greater equity, greater user satisfaction and lower costs for health systems has been demonstrated by countries in Europe, Canada and New Zealand, countries that have a universalising and inclusive health system, with principles similar to ours, such as: first contact, coordination, comprehensiveness and longitudinality. In addition, PHC is on the political agenda of these governments, in contradiction to the well-known fragmented, overspecialised health systems with excessive use of medical technologies. [1]

In Great Britain, in the 17th century, and officially in the last quarter of the 18th century, an alternative type of institution to the secular hospital was created, the so-called dispensary, which provided care for children, home care, including obstetric care and mainly for the poorer population. [1]

The differentiation of health services into three levels of care, primary, secondary and teaching, which is the basis for contemporary regionalised and hierarchical care systems, was proposed in England in 1920 by Lord Dauson of Penn, the medical authority for the public health system, and it is through this differentiation that the PHC proposal has been implemented in many countries. [1]

4.6.2. The PSF in Brazil

The Family Health Strategy (ESF) was designed to reorient the care model by implementing multi-professional teams in strategic units, restructuring the provision of basic health services. The ESF is now the gateway to the entire public health system in Brazil.

The state of Ceará is considered to be the birthplace of the Community Health Agents Programme (PACS) and played an important and decisive role in the implementation of the PSF in Brazil. Initially, the programme operated with money from the federal government's special emergency funds, and its work basically focused on providing guidance to the families assisted by these agents, who had previously undergone a two-week training course to increase their knowledge of health, with a view mainly to reducing infant mortality. [27]

Even before the experience in Ceará, there were proposals similar to the PSF in other Brazilian municipalities, such as the pioneering experiences in Porto Alegre (Vila de São José do Murialdo), still in the 1970s, and in the state of São Paulo. It should not be forgotten that similar programmes have been implemented in countless Brazilian municipalities, such as Niterói, Campinas, Londrina and others. [1]

We can't fail to emphasise the experience of the Family Doctor at the São Paulo State Health Department, which was short-lived and apparently left few local marks, but which was important, according to one interlocutor (SANTOS, 2002), for having opened the door to broadening the discussion about family medicine and primary health care in Brazil. In the second half of the 1980s, the Secretary of Health for the state of São Paulo, José Aristodemo Pinotti, first proposed the Cuban model of family medicine.

According to GOULART (2002)

> **The programme was widely criticised at the time, both from the right and the left (SANTOS, 2002). On the one hand, the powerful**
>
> **Paulista de Medicina, suspicious of the left-wing nature that could be brought about by an idea generated in Cuba; on the other, the Doctors' Union, denouncing its palliative or basket case nature. Within the health movement itself at the time, i.e. in national organisations such as CEBES and ABRASCO, or among municipal health secretaries, the project did not gain approval or penetration, remaining a marginal action to a certain extent.**

Perhaps, in view of what Goulart said, the PSF is still not widely accepted by many health professionals today. Perhaps this is a legacy of decades of discussions about a model of care that, at the time, did not have the results we have today to show how important and effective the Family Health Strategy is as a model of comprehensive care to be followed.

Some time later, in 1990, Law 8080, known as the Organic Health Law, and Law 8.142 were passed, defining the functioning of the SUS and supporting primary care as a priority for reorganising healthcare in Brazil.

In 1991, the Ministry of Health was enthusiastic about Ceará's successful experience and suggested the creation of the National Programme of Community Health Agents (PNAS), linked to the National Health Foundation (Funasa), which was first implemented in the Northeast and then in the North, with the main objective of helping to reduce infant mortality and maternal mortality. (VIANA and DAL POZ, 1998, p. 19) [27]

In 1992, called PACS, it was implemented through an agreement between Funasa/MS and the State Health Secretariats, with the provision of funds to fund the programme and the payment, in the form of a grant, of one minimum **monthly** wage **to the agents. With PACS,** "the focus **began to be on the** family as the unit of health programme action and no longer (just) the individual, and the notion of coverage area (**per family**) was introduced" **(VIANA; Dal POZ, 1998, p. 19).** [27]

In 1993, PACS covered 13 states in the North and Northeast regions, with 29,000 CHAs working in 761 municipalities. By November 1994, the programme was already operating in 987 municipalities in 17 states in the North, Northeast and Centre-West regions, with a total of 33,488 agents. [27]

Experiences such as the Family Doctor Programme, which was developed from 1992 in Niterói (RJ), with a structure similar to the family medicine implemented in Cuba and with advice from Cuban technicians, also influenced the Ministry of Health's decision in 1993 to create the Family Health Programme (PSF) which, like PACS, was institutionally linked to the Community Health Coordination (Cosac) in the National Health Foundation's Operations Department. [27, 19]

In September 1994, the Ministry of Health released the first document on the PSF, defining the agreement between the Ministry of Health, states and municipalities, with the funding mechanism, counterpart requirements and criteria for selecting municipalities. There were some requirements for the agreement to be signed, such as the functioning of both the Municipal Health Council and the Municipal Health Fund. The Family Health Programme was created to direct the organisation of healthcare, which from then on began to be municipalised. [27,5]

The PSF was not initially intended to replace the PACS and its implementation was aimed at areas of greater social risk, special areas registered by the government. [27]

In 1995, PACS and PSF were transferred from the National Health Foundation to the Secretariat of Health Care (SAS), and remained there until early 1999, when the programmes again changed institutional location to the Coordination of Primary Care of the Secretariat of Health Policies (SPS). [27]

In January 1996, the PSF began to be remunerated according to the SIA/SUS table of procedures, but at double the cost of the SUS consultation. In the 1997 and 1998 documents, the PSF was presented as a proposal to reorient the care model based on Primary Care, in accordance with the principles of the Unified Health System (SUS). [27]

Concerned to avoid the imminent pulverisation of the PSF, which would have a low impact and little resolution for the population, in November 1999 the Ministry of Health readjusted the transfer values and introduced a new method for calculating the financial incentives of the variable PAB for the PSF, paying more to municipalities with higher population coverage of the ESF. By May 2000, municipalities with coverage of at least 70% of their population had grown by 42%.[27]

By December 2002, the programme had 16,698 teams serving 55 million people, 31.8% of the population in 4,168 municipalities. The programme reached 83% of its target for the year. Compared to 2001, there was a 25 per cent increase in coverage. [27]

In the early years of the creation of the PSF, there was a difference, as mentioned above, in the amounts paid to PSF professionals, which were higher than those mentioned by the municipal secretariats themselves.

The Normative Evaluation of the PSF carried out in 2001 and 2003 led to a series of disqualifications of teams that were receiving funds from the Ministry of Health, but were working with irregularities, such as incomplete teams, lack of infrastructure for work, and failure by professionals to work 40 hours a day. The conditions under which professionals were hired were precarious (not statutory, not CLT), not guaranteeing that they would remain with the team for a long period of time, as well as exposing the contractor to the risk of labour lawsuits, and there was little involvement of professionals with the population in the first two years of work. Another weakness was the lack of participation by these professionals in training and development courses.

In 2007, a total of 27,324 PSF teams were set up in 5,125 municipalities, covering 46.6% of the Brazilian population, which corresponds to around 87.7 million people. There are 211,000 Community Health Agents in a total of 5,300 municipalities, covering 56.8 per cent of the Brazilian population, which corresponds to 107 million people. This year, R$4,064.00 million was invested in the programme.

Despite the good figures achieved (physical and financial), almost 15 years after the birth of the PSF in Brazil, the challenge remains, as there are still several limiting factors that need to be resolved: low integration capacity between PSF teams and teams from traditional primary care units and between the PSF teams themselves; the SIAB has been used in a limited and bureaucratic way, compromising the evaluation and monitoring of primary care actions; the lack of a referral and counter-referral system that guarantees continuity and integrality of health care; low capacity of PSF teams to draw up plans, projects, programmes and ongoing actions that enhance their relations with other sectors of government and society.

4.6.3. The PSF in the Federal District

The following account comes from one of the authors of this article, who went through this process as a nurse in a family health team.

The PSF in the Federal District has a history full of impasses, political interests (and disinterests), which culminated in its implementation and termination three times. The first time was during Cristóvam Buarque's administration in 1998, when the PSF was called "Saúde em Casa" (Health at Home). It was a great endeavour, with high coverage and teams that were almost always full, the population was very receptive to it, and even today they are calling for the return of "Saúde em Casa" (Health at Home). Due to political problems, this programme was discontinued, and with the arrival of a new government in 2002, the PSF was resumed by the State Health Department hiring the Candango Solidarity Institute (ICS) to manage the programme. However, the professionals were not selected, there were many political appointments and turnover was high, which culminated in the ICS being denounced to the Public Prosecutor's Office for administrative impropriety. As a result, the institute was investigated and the PSF was extinguished once again, suddenly leaving all the professionals unemployed overnight, and without any constitutional worker's rights guaranteed.

In 2003, the Zerbini Foundation (FZ) won a public tender to manage the PSF, which was renamed the "Healthy Family Programme", launched by the Roriz government in its third term. Some satellite towns were prioritised with greater team coverage, such as São Sebastião, which was in the throes of a Hantavirus epidemic. However, in most of the towns, the teams were spread out, generating low coverage and little impact on the health of the population in general, not reducing the demand for emergency care at the Regional Hospitals, which was a primary objective of the SES. Another strategy adopted by the Zerbini Foundation in conjunction with the SES-DF was the implementation of PACS in Health Centres.

This strategy was initially poorly accepted by the staff of the traditional health centres and by the population, due to the fact that it was not very effective, as it did not have a doctor. It was then suggested that an expanded PACS be created, which would have a doctor, as well as a nurse and CHAs, to improve care for the population in the catchment area. However, this project was gradually abandoned due to operational difficulties, since the Health Centres themselves, in which the PACS were located, didn't have enough doctors to meet the demand, and the PACS didn't cover the entire area of the Health Centre, so the PACS doctor could only see patients from his area of coverage, which led to conflicts with patients from other areas. In addition, the doctors from these teams gradually left, transforming the teams into ordinary PACS once again. In any case, the Zerbini Foundation managed the teams that were in place well, but once again there were accusations in the Public Prosecutor's Office of misappropriation of funds, salary delays occurred, and several demonstrations by the team's professionals also took place during this period. Although the FZ tried to defend itself against the accusations by proving that some of them were false, the MPDF began to demand of the SES-DF that it should assume its role as manager of the programme and should not renew the contract with the FZ, which expired in 2005, was extended for a year and would expire again in September 2006. The SES-DF then, in the midst of the accusations against FZ, did not renew the contract and all the professionals working on the Healthy Family Programme were fired, only this time with all their rights guaranteed. However, so that the programme wouldn't grind to a halt, those professionals who were from the SHS-DF and the FZ were given the choice of working in their place of origin or in the programme, and many went to the PSF, but there were still too few of them in relation to the number of teams. So, due to their experience in leading family health teams, many professionals who were from the FZ were hired by the SES-DF under the CLT regime, which generated a lot of controversy, especially among nurses, as there was a huge list of candidates to be called up. All the CHAs were kept working under Constitutional Amendment No. 51 and District Law No. 3,716 of 09/12/2005, amended by District Law No. 3,870 of 16/06/2006.

After all these impasses, to make matters worse for the Family Health Strategy in the Federal District, there was a major political transition, with the change of governor in 2007, and as usual, all the senior positions were removed, but new appointments were slow in coming, and there were several changes in the primary care directorate, making it difficult for the regional managers and the teams to carry out their work, since there was little support. It wasn't until December 2007 that a new directorate took over, bringing prospects for the implementation of the Family Health Programme.

4.6.4. The PSF in Samambaia

According to the Samambaia Regional Administration, this is a satellite city of the Federal District that was born with the intention of housing the high number of people who migrated from other parts of the country to the Federal District between 1989 and 1994. [a]In order to create an urban structure for these residents, on 25 October 1989 the city was officially created through Law 49 and Decree 11.291, making it the 12th Administrative Region of the Federal District - RA XII.

The urban planning project for the area, however, was born 11 years earlier. The Plano Estrutural de Organização Territorial (Peot), drawn up in 1978, already included the **"Samambaia - preliminary study"** project, **which was officially implemented in 1982. The first plots in the city were** sold in quadra 406 and in the Setor de Mansões Leste (now Taguatinga). As early as 1985, the first residents began living in the city.

Three years after the first occupations, 3,381 houses were built for low-income families, mainly civil servants. The homes were purchased with the support of the Social Interest Housing System (SHIS), financed by the National Bank.

Between 1989 and 1992, the city experienced population swelling with the arrival of a large mass of residents, generally poor families, who received plots in semi-urbanised areas under the "concession of use system".

The region comprises urban and rural areas. The urban area is divided into the North and South sectors. The rural part is made up of the Guariroba Isolated Area and the Tabatinga Rural Nucleus. In 1996, the East Mansion Sector (SML) was dismembered from Samambaia and became part of the city of Taguatinga.

Population characteristics: In 2006, according to data from DIVAL, the population was 181,000. And according to the Samambaia Regional Administration, in 2007 the population already exceeded 203,000. However, all the surveys carried out by the Ministry of Health are based on the IBGE, which in 2006 had a population of just over 170,000. These population differences even make it difficult to organise the structure of the Family Health Strategy for the region.

In terms of migration, most of the population (72,484 inhabitants) was born in the Federal District. There is also a strong contingent of northeasterners (45,384 people) and migrants from the Southeast: 14,475 people. In terms of colour, 38,256 people declared themselves to be white, 4,734 black, 1,687 yellow, 65,083 mulatto, 463 indigenous and 37,684 did not declare.

In terms of health care, Samambaia has a Regional Hospital with 142 beds, six of which are not accredited and are ICU beds. It was bought by the GDF in 2003 and was previously a private hospital. For this reason, it has a smaller physical structure that differs from the other public hospitals in the Federal District. Initially bed occupancy was 30 per cent and today it is at 66 per cent. This Regional also has 4 Health Centres, three of which cover an average of 70,000 inhabitants, and one, which is the Centre that is the subject of this study, covers more than 13,000 inhabitants, in both urban and rural areas.

The director of the Samambaia Regional Health Department, in office in 2006, observing the population's deficient primary health care, with a small number of basic units in relation to the population, a shortage of professionals, especially doctors, in the basic units, the under-utilisation of nurses' work, the overcrowding of the newly opened emergency room, and also his knowledge of the philosophy of the family health strategy, including in countries such as England, and the opportunity at that time to have a competition for community health doctors and nurses, In addition, his knowledge of the philosophy of the family health strategy, including that of other countries such as England, and the fact that at that time there was a competition for community health doctors and nurses, motivated him to seek the implantation and implementation of the PSF in Samambaia, and the conversion of Health Centre No. 03.

It was then that, in contact with the central level of the SES/DF, this implementation was articulated, since it was an initiative of the SES/DF, since there was already interest in taking this initiative to restructure primary care.

The aim of better primary care was to control chronic diseases such as hypertension and diabetes, reduce the rate of child malnutrition, reduce the number of hospitalisations of children under five due to preventable diseases, reduce the incidence of cervical cancer, reduce the number of women over 30 who had never had preventive care, offer a greater number of prenatal consultations and increase the uptake of respiratory symptoms.

The second and no less important objective of implementing the strategy in the regional centre is to reduce demand on the emergency department, avoiding cases that should be dealt with at primary level, which account for the vast majority of emergency department visits at this hospital.

In 2006, Samambaia had three family health teams (ESF) in isolated units (a rented house, one provided by the Regional Administration and one owned by the SES), three PACS teams in the three oldest and most traditional Health Centres, and a further three ESF teams in Health Centre No. 03, which changed its organisational structure from traditional to family health.

In 2008, with the hiring of new professionals, the process of converting the other Health Centres in Samambaia, which already had CHWs because of the PACS, began, and they received doctors, nurses and nursing technicians to set up new teams and extinguish the PACS. However, this process was not fully completed due to the lack of physical space for all the new teams to work in. As a result, the managers of each Health Centre made adaptations that they considered most suitable for the professionals to work in, and to this day they are waiting for units to be built or rented for these teams to work in. It's worth pointing out that many of them are already incomplete due to doctor turnover.

4.6.5. The PSF at Samambaia Health Centre No. 03

Health Centre No. 03 is Samambaia's newest health centre, inaugurated on 14 December 1999 to meet the demand of this expansion area, which until June 2008 had 13,960 inhabitants, 12,978 in the urban area and 679 in the rural area. Since then, however, the Federal District government has built a settlement for needy families living in risky areas, and they have gradually been transferred to this new area, where the regional administration has created more blocks to urbanise and organise the new housing in a regularised way. As a result, the population of the expansion has increased to around 10,000 inhabitants, according to the Regional Administration, and the population of the Health Centre No. 03 area has increased to almost 24,000 people. In other words, the population has almost doubled, and this has caused major problems for the operation of the Family Health Strategy at the health centre in question. The Health Centre area has two primary schools, two nurseries, a community centre, several churches and a small local business.

In December 2009, the workforce was made up as follows:

Professional/ Position	Workload	Quantity	Workload	Quantity
	Before the Conversion (2006)		After the Conversion (2009)	
Manager	40	01	40	01
Head of the Nursing Centre	40	01	40	01
Head of the Operational Support Centre (NAO)	40	01	40	01
Head of the Regulation, Control and Evaluation Centre (NRCA)	40	01	40	01
Gynaecologist	40	01	40	01
Medical clinic	40	01	-	-
Paediatrician	20	02	15	01
Nurse	40	01	40	05
	20	-	20	01
General Practitioners	-	-	40	03
Social Worker	40	01	-	-
Female dentists	40	02	40	01
	20	-	20	01
Nursing assistants	40	09	40	15
	30	01	20	02
Laboratory assistants	40	01	40	01
	30	01	30	-
Social work assistant	40	01	40	01
Administrative assistants	40	03	40	06
	30	03	30	01

The Health Centre functioned in its traditional model, with the programmes recommended by the SES/FD, consisting of a reception room for children, women and adults, a tuberculosis programme room, a dressing room, a vaccination room, a medication and nebulisation room, five doctors' offices, two dental offices with a brushing room, a dispensing pharmacy and an internal pharmacy, a laboratory collection point, a storeroom, a CHA room and a meeting room. In addition, there was an administrative structure, with a filing cabinet, rooms for the manager and heads of nursing and operational support.

The 03 Samambaia Health Centre was selected as a pilot project by the Federal District government to implement a new model of primary care where the traditional model would be replaced by the Ministry of Health's Family Health Strategy.

The choice of the primary care unit that would be converted into a PSF was made at a workshop held in the first half of 2006 with the participation of members of the central level (SES-DF), some members of FEPECS, representatives of the central and regional managers of the Family Health Programme in force at the time and the management of some regional health centres, including Samambaia. This workshop decided on Samambaia Health Centre 3 on the grounds that it was geographically located in a well-defined area, with a population close to the Ministry of Health's standard for setting up three FHP teams, had a physical structure that needed little adaptation and had a PACS operating with 10 CHWs.

The routine of care was also traditional, with the scheduling of programmes, as described below:

Growth and Development Programme (CD): after an educational meeting, the paediatricians were scheduled for medical appointments, with two first CDs, six return visits, two emergency appointments and 10 tickets for spontaneous demand.

Prenatal care programme: the card was opened by the nursing assistants, and the first medical appointment with the gynaecologist was scheduled; after the medical appointment, educational meetings were scheduled by the nurse, interspersed with these medical appointments.

Family Planning Programme: this was an open agenda, with 20 places. First there was a meeting and then the gynaecologist saw the patients in individual consultations.

Hypertensive and Diabetic Programme: patients who arrived were booked into the medical clinic for diagnosis, or if they arrived with proof of diagnosis, they were booked in with the nurse for the group, after which they were booked in for a medical consultation. The meetings for each patient took place every three months, as did the consultations. In the clinic's diary, there were 20 hours a week to attend to hypertensive and diabetic patients and the nurse had weekly appointments, but in order to meet all the demand, patients came every three months. The other 20 hours were for general practice, where the elderly and those with special needs were booked. This schedule was half open with a password and half by appointment. These groups were unsuccessful because there were many absences and little involvement on the part of the staff and it was impossible to actively seek them out.

Tuberculosis and leprosy programme: open agenda, no specific day, carried out by trained professionals.

Dentistry: attended to the zero caries, hypertensive and diabetic and prenatal programmes, with educational talks and clinical care. There were no dental assistants or dental hygiene technicians. They rely on the support of the nursing team to prepare and sterilise their equipment. The dentists themselves do all the appointments, including booking appointments and door-to-door services.

The NRCA was the same as the entire network, with medical records separated by date of birth, and was responsible for retrieving and filing medical records, attaching exams, and scheduling outpatient speciality clinics in the network, as well as productivity statistics.

Procedure room: spontaneous demand.

Vaccination room and heel prick test: spontaneous demand, as recommended by the Ministry of Health.

The assistants' schedules were rotated and prioritised according to each assistant's profile and vaccination training.

As already mentioned, there was also the **PACS,** with 10 CHWs, who made home visits under the supervision of a nurse, and had a room to carry out their administrative activities.

With the new work proposal, the unit, which used to have a paediatrician, general practitioner and gynaecologist, now has general practitioners, a nursing team and community health workers.

The nurses' work was limited to educational talks on family planning, growth and development and prenatal care, the tuberculosis programme and the coordination of this programme.

The lack of a model to serve as a source of research was the biggest difficulty in implementing this new type of care, as the unit that emerged was no longer a health centre, but neither was it a PSF unit.

The first step was, as described above, choosing the unit, territorialisation and mapping of the catchment area.

The next step was to register the teams and update the National Code of Health Establishments (CNES), which included the new professionals (doctors and nurses) and those already working in the unit.

The model implemented kept some of the activities of the traditional health centre, such as booking specialities, imaging tests, attendance statistics, laboratory, pharmacy and immunobiological room, and added activities exclusive to the PSF, such as home visits by different professionals from the unit, specific statistics - production reports and markers for evaluation.

Three teams were set up in the new structure. A general practitioner and a nurse were hired for each team. Three nursing technicians from the unit itself were chosen by the managers according to their profile for the teams, and the ten community health agents who were from the Zerbini Foundation, and from that moment on had an employment contract with the SES/FD, due to the end of their contract, were distributed to the three teams.

At first, triage by clinic (adult, women's and children's rooms) was maintained, with the nursing assistant in each room carrying out triage for the three new teams, both for medical and nursing care, and from the moment of triage the patient was directed to the doctor or nurse in their team. This was a very tumultuous period in the unit, as the same server controlled a large number of appointments, leading to confusion and delays. What's more, this form of reception didn't allow the initial care professionals to form a bond with the families.

In this initial transition phase, the specialists were kept, which generated a great deal of conflict in terms of care, including duplication of care, because patients who were used to being seen by the traditional model didn't accept being seen only by the **general practitioner. According to the manager, patients said they "wanted their child's paediatrician", or only trusted their gynaecologist, and didn't** understand that only one doctor could see both mother and child. The nursing consultation was also difficult to accept at first, as it was a procedure unknown to this population.

Since the family health strategy model of care required the team to have a total bond with the population, the reception rooms for children, women and adults were transformed into a team reception room, where triage was carried out for all types of care. The room was set up with a scale for adults, a digital scale for children, an anthropometric table, a tensiometer, a tape measure and forms for all the programmes.

Each room was labelled with the team number, the catchment area and the names of its members. A standard colour was adopted to identify each room. The catchment area was also publicised to the population by means of a banner displayed outside the Health Centre. Gradually the population became orientated as to which team they belonged to, accepted the new model of care and showed satisfaction with the care provided by the general practitioner and the nurse. As a result, there was a significant drop in the productivity of the specialist doctors, justifying their removal to other units. However, the high demand for medical clinic patients and the presence of a significant portion of the population living in the rural area, which is not covered by the PSF and belongs to the area covered by this Health Centre, meant that the General Practitioner had to continue to provide 20 hours of care.

The CHAs played an important role in informing the population about the new care model. As well as providing information at home, they orientated patients arriving at the unit as to the flow to be followed, helped to identify out-of-area patients and integrated very satisfactorily with the new teams.

At one point there was a temporary change in the area covered by Centre 3, which took over some blocks that belonged to Health Centre 2 due to administrative problems at that unit. This population was redistributed between the teams, exceeding the limit of the number of families to be assisted. This went on for around three months and caused a great deal of disruption to the progress of the work, since the professionals were unable to provide adequate care, the area was physically remote, which made home visits difficult, and the CHAs were assigned to Centre No. 2.
Once the negative results of this change had been verified, the original catchment area was returned.

Consecutive changes in a short space of time, demands for standardisation from society and the civil servants themselves generated a high level of stress in the teams, which was accompanied by an increase in the number of absences. There were personal conflicts, but they were gradually resolved.

Every change generates fear and anguish, which was aggravated by the lack of training, especially for the nursing technicians, who didn't take the introductory PSF course or any other training that covered the programme's philosophy. Doctors and nurses, on the other hand, have been favoured with a large number of courses, but this has led to numerous rescheduled appointments for these professionals.

The unit's Regulation, Control and Evaluation Centre (NRCA), which had seven employees at the start of the conversion, was reduced to just three, which caused a number of problems such as delays in filing exams and medical records, forwarding medical records and appointments for speciality care and even for in-house care. It also caused delays in the delivery of productivity statistics. It remained closed for external services for over a year.

The nursing procedures carried out in the Health Centre were a major point of conflict with the PSF regulations, since in the PSF the nursing technician of each team carries out all the procedures for their team, such as screening, glycaemia, dressing, BP measurement, nebulisation, vaccination, etc... However, as the unit in question is large and now houses three family health teams in the same physical space, it has not been possible to adjust these procedures to how they would work in a unit with just one team. Attempts were made with glycaemia, where the nursing technician who was in triage would be doing this procedure, but it didn't work because the booked patients began to complain that those who came in to do glycaemia were being passed over, and patients who were fasting to do the test also complained because they were waiting a long time to be seen.

The demand for basic specialities was an initial concern for the general practitioners and the Health Centre managers, as it was thought that they would have many difficulties, especially with paediatrics and gynaecology, due to their non-specialist training. Initially, there was a greater demand for paediatrics, but the centre had the support of the manager, who was a paediatrician. Gradually, the difficulties encountered by the generalists were resolved and, over time, this demand decreased dramatically, to the point where the generalists needed less support from the paediatrician.

As far as gynaecology is concerned, at the beginning we managed to negotiate with the regional management for a gynaecologist for five hours a week to meet the demand of patients referred by the general practitioner and the nurses, and after two years of conversion we managed to get a 40-hour gynaecologist for the unit.

Three years after the conversion of the care model, both patients and staff have already adapted.

The nurses' services were expanded to include individual consultations in outpatient nursing clinics for the various programmes run by the Federal District's Health Department and the Ministry of Health, such as CD consultations, prenatal consultations, consultations with hypertensive and diabetic patients, home visits, consultations for the tuberculosis programme, STD/AIDS consultations, consultations for the leprosy programme, diabetic foot assessments, hypertension and diabetes groups, family planning and prenatal consultations. In addition, gynaecology consultations for the collection of oncotic cytology were also carried out by the nurses, even with the presence of a gynaecologist.

According to the head of nursing, after the conversion the demand for prenatal care fell a lot, due to the greater control of only seeing patients who live in the area, as the demand from outside was very high.

In February 2008, doctors and nurses from the three teams were trained in the rapid test for HIV diagnosis, which was implemented in the Samambaia Regional Office as a pilot in the Federal District, and everyone took on this role, which has been positive for patients, especially pregnant women, who now have the results in good time to take the necessary precautions.

Patients have got used to being divided into teams according to address. They already go to the general practitioner and the nurses, they like the appointments, and they no longer complain that they wanted the paediatrician or the gynaecologist. As a result, the bond with the unit and the professional has intensified, and the patient has come to know the professionals responsible for their care, making it easier to solve their problems and access the service. However, with the new settlements, this peace of mind has come to an end, as demand has increased greatly and the clinic has been lost, which has made access even more difficult.

Currently, appointments are made for each professional in the teams, with half of the patients booked and the other half from the spontaneous demand agenda, checking each patient's priorities. There is a weekly schedule of appointments,
as recommended by the PSF, where each professional has one type of service per period. As shown in the table below.

In order to draw up this rota, it is necessary to look at the availability of rooms, since there isn't a consulting room for each nurse and doctor, as we only have five consulting rooms. In addition, it is necessary to ensure the constant presence of the doctor or nurse from each team at the Health Centre, in order to resolve any problems their team may have. It is also necessary to have at least one doctor present at any given time, in order to avoid the problem of there being no doctor at the Health Centre in the event of an emergency, which leads to little satisfaction on the part of users, who often don't understand, when it isn't an emergency, why they can't be seen if there is a doctor at the unit, since when this happens, the doctor who stays on usually already has his own appointments.

Morning	Mon	Have	Wed	Here	Sex
E 07	Doctor E 7 Group		Doctor E 7 Group	Doctor E 7 Paediatrics	Nurse E 7 CD
E 09	Paediatrician	Doctor E 9 Paediatrics	Doctor E 9 Pre-Christmas	Nurse E 9 EC	Doctor E G G
E 10	Doctor E 10 Pre-Christmas	Doctor E 10 Paediatrics	Nurse E 7 EC	Doctor E 9 G	Doctor E 10 G
cco	Nurse E 9	Nurse E 7	Nurse E10	Nurse E10 PN	
CM	Clinic	Paediatrician		Clinic	Clinic
R. Ed.		Nurse E 9			Nurse E10
VD		Nurse E10 Doctor E 7	Nurse E 9 Doctor E 10	Doctor E 10 Nurse E 7	Nurse E 9 Doctor E 7
Afternoon	Mon	Have	Wed	Here	Sex
E 07	Doctor E 7 Paediatrics	Doctor E 7 CM	Nurse E 7 PN	Doctor E 7	
E 09	Nurse E 9 PN	Nurse E 9 CD		Doctor E 9 Paediatrics	Doctor E 9 CM
E 10	Doctor E 10 CM	Nurse E10 CD	Doctor E 10 PED	Nurse E10 CE	Doctor E 10 G
CCO				Gynaecologist	Nurse E 7
CM			Clinic	Paediatrician	
R. Ed.	ODONTO	Nurse E 7	Nurse E 9	Nurse E 7	Nurse E10
VD		Doctor E 9	Doctor E 9 Nurse E10		Nurse E 7

booked patients and only takes emergency cases from the other teams.

Currently, some nursing procedures are centralised in order to speed up patient care. Thus, blood glucose, nebulisation, medication and dressings are the responsibility of a trained nursing technician and vaccinations are the responsibility of another trained technician, where these procedures are carried out by all the teams.

In each team's reception room, scheduled patients are triaged, and spontaneous demand is received and referred as necessary, according to each patient's health priorities. It is also in this room that the pre-natal card is opened, initial care is given to those with respiratory symptoms, medical records are reviewed with an active search for notifications, appointments are booked, patients are advised on the flow of this health unit, active listening is carried out and the Bolsa Família is monitored.

The nursing technicians were divided into three teams, one with four and the others with three. The roster is made according to the profile and training of each one. Other technicians are assigned to vaccination, dressing and medication, epidemiological surveillance and the CME (sterile material centre).

The laboratory, pharmacy and storeroom remained with the same service routine, as there was no need for changes. However, a computerised system was implemented for dispensing medicines and materials, both in the pharmacy and the storeroom.

The release of medication for patients was also computerised through the implementation of the Citizen's Health Card, the same card that was already being used to computerise the entire network, and the electronic medical record, which was implemented throughout the Samambaia Regional Health Centre, where Health Centre No. 03 was the first to be implemented, which generated another period of turbulence for this unit, and which was the subject of several comments from staff during the data collection of this research.

After a long period with its activities limited, the NRCA was given a new head, who gradually and quickly managed to organise the filing of medical records and exams, speciality appointments, the structure of the archive and even began to serve the public every day in the morning for speciality appointments. All this with the existing staff of three, and it was only possible because of the hard work and, in particular, the computerisation of the unit, which made it possible not to have to pick up medical records every day for appointments.

Finally, as a supplementary activity, self-massage was introduced in the first half of 2009 by a nursing technician who had been trained to do it. The activities take place twice a week for elderly patients and the hypertensive and diabetic groups.

CHAPTER 5

Discussion

5.1. Interviews

5.1.1. Staff perception of improved patient care with conversion

The improvement in the population's health care is visible and widely reported by those who have experienced the traditional model and started working in the new model, the family health strategy.

In order for primary care to be of high quality, it is necessary to have professionals who are responsible and committed to the community, which is why it is often said that professionals who work in the ESF must have the right profile to work in this strategy. [11]

According to CONASS (2007), every encounter between one or more health professionals and a user or family should be welcoming, friendly, promote autonomy and empowerment, and be characterised by mutual trust by including the user in the process of their own care. As one of the unit's employees put it

> **"It created a** greater **bond** between professionals and the community. When it was just a health centre, the professional didn't have a bond with the patient. Whoever you saw **came in, left their complaint and left"**

The family and the environment in which it lives and is inserted is the main focus of the PSF, whose mission is to establish links with this population, hence the need for the ACS to live in the community in which they work, as they know the area, the residents, the problems experienced there and become the main link between the team and the community, so that co-responsibility for the population's health is created. [2]

The issue of the bond is recurrent in the speeches and shows us how important this is for the health of the population, because the bond empowers the professional to act more precisely, but it also brings difficulties to the day-to-day work insofar as the patient demands more from the professional precisely because there is this bond, and the professional feels obliged to offer feedback to the patient, which is not always possible due to the difficulties experienced in the health unit, such as the high demand, which far exceeds what is stipulated by the Ministry of Health.

> **"The positive thing I think is that we get to work with the patient, their family and get to** know them well. I like this integration. We don't just provide guidance, we get to know the conditions in which these patients live, so we can adapt to them too. We have a bond with them, a kind of family bond. We make money to help buy **filters and food. We do bazaars, everything, fairs, etc."**
>
> **"the volume of sick leave has increased because professionals are getting sicker in** this new model

as they are more involved with their families and their problems, and the demand for **services has increased a lot."**

The resolvability of patients' problems was also reported by the professionals, because by working with the new model it is possible to get to know the patient as a whole, to find out about their complaints, from gynaecological to clinical, in a single consultation. This makes it easier to offer a solution to their health problems, and it is also possible to get feedback on whether the proposed treatment was followed and whether there was a good therapeutic response, since the CHWs visit the patients on a monthly basis and provide this feedback to the team. This is clear from the following statements:

> "Resolubility has improved. Now we can give feedback to the **population."**

> **"When you go into people's homes, you start to see** socio-economic issues, cultural issues, family members, and that makes it easier for you to provide care and conduct yourself. When you provide care, you know that there are certain **guidelines that there's no point in giving if people haven't done them. So that makes it much easier"**

> **"I think that together with the team we can** solve more of the **patient**'s problems **today."**

> **"Because the number of doctors has increased, (...) because the doctors are** general practitioners, they don't just treat you as a doctor, just as a gynaecologist, they treat you as a whole, you know? So it's better for the patient, instead of having to make an appointment with a gynaecologist or a doctor, they just make an appointment and it **solves their problem, you know? It was good in that respect."**

In the specific case of the PSF, it can be seen that its implementation, in technical and political terms, is being proposed and/or carried out on the basis of interaction with the community, with the aim of building more effective practices and strategies for tackling health problems in a participatory way.[12]

> **"I mean, we end up getting to know them better** because the PSF is about **getting to know the patient, their family, their environment and everything."**

> **"There was a closer relationship with the community."**

In the technical sense, the PSF needs to be the gateway to the system with a health practice that incorporates traditional medical care into a logic that is effectively health promotion. Without these changes, the proposal could remain just a talking point and fail to bring about the changes it propagates[13] . Health promotion and prevention are well understood by professionals as an essential part of the actions carried out by family health teams:

> **"Another thing is that the preventive part has improved,** because that's where we **work most with the community."**

However, there are several obstacles to the implementation of this key part of the strategy, such as the high demand in the Health Centre area and the Health Department's requirement that doctors must see 20 patients in a five-hour period, which is a recurring complaint of these professionals, who report the difficulty of carrying out a proper consultation, looking not only at the patient's main complaint, but also at secondary complaints, the way of life that may influence this complaint, individual and collective habits, among others. To see all this, 15 minutes of consultation is insufficient in most cases to achieve quality care and to be able to address prevention and health promotion.

In view of this, the work of the nurse comes into play a lot, as they are obliged to attend a slightly smaller number of appointments and can work more on health promotion, guiding patients to avoid simple problems that could bring them back to the unit in a short time if they don't receive this guidance.

Improving access was mentioned a lot by the professionals, as the daily open and closed agenda was fundamental to improving access. The closed agenda works for patients from specific population groups such as pregnant women, children under six, hypertensive and diabetic patients, women for oncotic cytology collection, and the open agenda works for patients with complaints, the main ones observed being: fever, colds and flu, throat infection, decompensated hypertensive and diabetic patients, skin conditions and respiratory allergies. The following verbalisations illustrate this improvement:

> **"The ease both of getting there and of getting what you want."**

> **"I believe that patients have found it easier to** book appointments, more access and also the issue of patients being able to book appointments and not wait **too long."**

There are professionals who report the difficulty they experience in terms of access, because it's clear that it has improved, but there are many complaints from patients about delays, both in receiving care and in making appointments, and this is a cause of suffering for the professionals who work at the front door - the nursing technicians. Some CHAs also complain for the same reason, and suffer from this complaint from patients.

> **"I think** the population **should value** this and they don't, I don't see many difficulties in getting appointments or tests, because I have a health insurance plan, I pay a lot and I get an appointment every two months and here they get appointments overnight, the group didn't even come today (Friday) and the return is for Monday, in the private sector this doesn't **exist, you know."**

Comprehensive care, set out by both the Ministry of Health and the Federal Constitution itself, as one of the guidelines of the SUS and also of the family health strategy, appears in the verbalisations of the civil servants as one of the major improvements that have occurred with the conversion, since patients are no longer seen only as a complaint and are now seen as a whole, integrated into a community, and surrounded by family members and an environment with which they interact and which can interfere with their health. As a result, patient care became more humanised.

> **"[Care] has become more targeted,** so only that doctor sees that patient, so the doctor knows more about what they're dealing with and the patient doesn't have to start from scratch when they have

to see the doctor again because of their **history."**

"The positive points are that the population has more **access, you know, to** certain programmes, for example, hypertensive patients are monitored, they don't keep changing doctors, each one gives them a different medicine, you don't know, I mean, we end up **getting to** know them **better** because the PSF is about getting to know the patient, their family, their environment and everything."

"The service has become **more humanised"**

The Community Health Agents (ACS) and home visits are strategic points of operation for the strategy. The CHWs are the community's link to the family health teams, they are the ones who are at patients' homes every day, bringing information and complaints and problems from the community, they are the ones who take patients to their scheduled appointments with specialists, they help the team with patient health education, they choose critical patients who need more care to be visited

by both the doctor and the nurse, showing yet another guideline of the programme, which is Equity. Home visits were also described by all the professionals, including, to our surprise, the doctors, as essential to the team's weekly routine. They don't give up on the visit, because through it they can get to know the community in which they work better, as well as solving the problems of patients who can't get to the health centre, or even patients who are resistant to treatment, who end up giving in and following the doctor's and nurse's recommendations, thus improving their quality of life. Not to mention the fact that doctors and nurses use the weekly visits to supervise the work of the CHWs, a very important function if the activities are to be carried out successfully and if all families are to be properly monitored. The speeches below illustrate the point:

"One of the positive things about the PSF is the agents, because they're inside the community, they see the situation, the problems in the community and they bring them to **us."**

"and z visit Z good, because they feel, Z, as they say, privileged, important when we go there, and we know the environment where they live, right. So it's **easier for you to deal with their illnesses, you know, deal with the situation."**

However, it was noted that in practice, home visits are once again somewhat hampered by excessive demand, as several times doctors have been prevented from leaving for visits because of the need to increase clinical care, or because of the lack of other doctors in the unit, due to their holidays, leaves or bonuses, or because of the need to carry out bureaucratic services.

The project has already demonstrated its potential as a social force for promoting change. Its introduction is seen in a positive light, as it has a substitutive character, proposing to introduce a new structuring axis for health services, capable of giving direction to changes in the care and organisational practices of the SUS. [13]

The structuring perspective of the FHP in the process of reorganising basic services in the SUS makes it possible to introduce organisational and operational innovations into the Municipal Health System[14] . There are discussions that recognise the notoriety of the Family Health Programme in Brazil, especially when it was institutionalised as a ministerial project.

5.1.2. Difficulties with conversion

The greatest difficulties encountered arose from the pioneering situation. With no model to follow and no prior training for employees, the conversion process became traumatic. Personal efforts and several attempts led to the creation of what is done today and many employees have already adapted to the new model, as the following verbalisations show:

> **"We didn't have a model to follow**. We had no technical support. We made a lot of mistakes, we had a lot of wear and tear, a lot of conflict. Sometimes it was one way, sometimes it **was another. One day we thought: I think this will work."**

> **"We tried** one way and it didn't work, so we tried another. We tried to organise the medication one way and it didn't work, so we went back and tried another way. I think this teamwork between all the teams is what made **the PSF work."**

> **"The lack of standardisation of services initially led to many conflicts."**

The population also had a period of adjustment; at first they complained a lot. The educational meetings were used to clarify the new way the health centre works and the new division into teams. Some still don't understand why they can't be seen by the doctor if he's there, just because he's not their doctor.

> **"And for the community it was something new**. When the community arrived and we said 'you **don't have to come here anymore, you have to come somewhere else', I spent about three months** using half of the educational meetings to explain what was going on, the **new way the health centre worked, to try and ease the stress."** AE1

> **"And sometimes the patient doesn't understand** much because sometimes there's a doctor from the other team and the one from your team isn't there, so they don't understand why they won't be seen **even though there is a doctor."**

These comments from the professionals show a little of the difficulty of having more than one team in the same unit, because, even though the Ministry of Health recommends in decree 648/2006 that professionals should work in and run a family health unit, it is not easy to work with many teams in the same physical space, because of the population's understanding of this, because of internal conflicts, such as different ways of working for each professional, who, even if they follow what is recommended to the letter, each has their own individual way of working in a team, of working in the various programmes that are carried out, and this ends up creating disagreements between the teams.

The professionals' distress at the way the conversion was carried out was a constant feature of their verbalisations. And the main reason for this suffering was the lack of training for the team to work in the new model, because as most of the professionals were former members of the unit, the Health Department didn't make the introductory course available to everyone, only new recruits were offered places on the course, most of them doctors and nurses, while the nursing technicians, who would undergo the biggest change to the way of working they were used to, didn't have the chance to go on the course. In addition, the unit's local managers, the Centre Manager and the Head of Nursing, also had no experience in the family health strategy, and from an outsider's point of view they were heroines, as they managed to completely change the way the unit worked, following what they heard about how family health should be and what the SES/DF demanded at local meetings. They also made use of the experience of the doctors and nurses who had already had experience of the strategy.

The training and continuing education of the teams is provided for in the National Primary Care Policy[4] , which sets a deadline of three months for the introductory course and makes the Federal District Health Department responsible for organising and offering this course and all the other continuing education courses necessary for the smooth running of the Strategy's activities. However, this was not prioritised at the time, as the following statements illustrate:

> **"What I think got in the way was that the officials weren't** prepared. So much so that they weren't even trained. To this day, some of them find it hard to accept, there are those who say it won't work. There was a lack of **training."**

> **"It's because we didn't have any kind of training,** we were simply **told 'Today it's a Health Centre, tomorrow it won't be any more, it's a PSF.** So the conversion happened overnight. And another thing is that there was no training, so it became a tumultuous thing, a more difficult thing, not now, now **everyone here is more adapted to the situation, but in the beginning it was horrible. Sad."**

There is currently a consensus, albeit partial, around the PSF proposal, with regard to the possibility of the programme being an operational instrument that can guarantee a change in the health practices of the SUS. The great controversy is over the scope of this strategy. In this sense, we can assimilate it as a **strategy that can bring about** change, where there are available resources that have not yet been utilised.

In this context, we realised that the changes imposed by the SES/DF for that health unit made it possible to break with an existing pattern of primary care in the Federal District that worked very well in the 1980s when it was created, but which deteriorated and there were no proposals for reform. The current ESF proposal brought hope of improvements, which did indeed materialise, but for this to happen, everyone had to go through a difficult and, for some, even traumatic process, which made it even more difficult to adapt to and accept the new way of working.

> **"Now for the employees it was horrible,** [laughs].... Because everything that's new brings a lot of frustration. We had no preparation, no support, they just came here and said, do it. And we had to do it the way we could, we tried various ways, until we found a way that worked. But now it's **smooth sailing."**

> **"I thought I wouldn't fit in.** But when I managed to settle in and show **my quality, then it was good."**

Depression, stress, confusion, suffering, tense, exhausting, were many adjectives used by civil servants to describe the conversion process

The following verbalisations show how difficult this process was:

> "**You have no idea how painful it** was to turn this place into a PSF, it was a war. Until the technicians understood that it was no longer a health centre, but a PSF, it was a long struggle. **Until the ACSs, who were from Zerbini,** understood that they were now from the secretariat and that we were going to work together, it was a struggle. It was fight after **fight. Very exhausting."**

> "**I think it's improved, now, more towards now, it's improved a lot, in the** beginning it was a bit **confusing,** they didn't know, now they don't, now **everyone's adapted, everyone knows, so it's easier."**

> "**Today, now that we've adapted, it's better, we feel a lighter atmosphere,** before it was very **tense."**

> "**The conversion for the patient I think was very** good, but for the staff I think it was **stressful."**

5.1.3. Influence of standardisation and management on strategy performance.

Management is key to the smooth running of a health unit, especially in the case of the Family Health Strategy, as it requires a lot of information, training of professionals and even the manipulation of statistical data that the Ministry of Health requires in order to maintain the transfer of funds to the Strategy.

At the health centre that is the subject of this study, there have been many problems with local management during the almost four years since the conversion process began. Firstly, as mentioned above, the managers responsible for the conversion did not receive adequate training to operationalise the necessary changes, and yet they managed to carry out this process successfully. After that, the manager of the Health Centre

left, and successive changes of management and departures of professionals began, which jeopardised the functioning of the unit. In addition, changes in the regional directorate were one of the factors that jeopardised the continuity of the actions implemented and developed by the Family Health Strategy. The following verbalisations demonstrate this:

> "**It's** become fashionable here now to change **heads** every day because of politics. And so someone starts a job, lays the foundations, things go along, the next thing you know, it's gone, another one comes along, with different ideas, and it starts all over again, you know? And we have to end up adapting to the way of working, so this leads to frustration **and indignation, and** there **end up being disagreements between employees"**

> "**The constant change of director** is also bad, because when you **adapt you change. A stone that rolls a lot doesn't create slime."**

The Federal District also has a particularity that hinders the development of full management, which is the fact that all investment is centralised, all financial control is done by the Central level, the Regionals, which are the satellite cities, do not have financial autonomy, and as a result everything from small repairs in the unit, such as changing a tap, to the purchase of supplies, depend on requests from the central level. And it's not just a lack of financial autonomy: the regional health centres have almost no autonomy, not even over the professionals they receive, who must be assigned according to what is defined at the central level of the SES/DF. The professionals realise these difficulties:

> **"Because it doesn't just depend on the person here, it depends on the** hospital, it depends on the routine, on delivering and bringing in material."

In addition, there was a lack of supervision and support from both the regional and central levels of the Primary Care Directorate. The only sector that is more present in the unit is the Monitoring and Evaluation Management, which is always in the unit and always in contact due to the implementation of the SIAB (Primary Care Information System) in the unit, which has been presenting problems in its execution since its implementation. The civil servants complain a lot about the lack of presence of the Regional Office and also about the fact that the central level has somewhat neglected the unit, which was initially targeted by the SES/DF as a model unit to be followed for the conversion of other units. However, this didn't happen, and the staff are quite vocal about this fact.

> "Whoever manages it, because the **regional centre** should **invest** more, you know? Because they know it's something that, in the future, the whole of Brazil will have, right? So it's something that's been implemented here. If it's established here, it has to continue here for things to move on elsewhere. **This should be the first place, the model."**

> **"There should at least be a meeting between the director of** GAPESF and all the PSF coordinators, and there isn't one! There's a general meeting at least once a month, so that they're aware of our difficulties. So there are lots of **difficulties, and this demotivates us."**

With regard to management, the professionals' biggest villain is quality versus quantity. The Department of Health demands quantity, with its own rules that recommend 20 medical consultations in a 5-hour period, and the professionals who want to work on prevention and promotion report not being able to do this part, which is a guideline of family health, due to the rules of the SES/DF. As a result, quality suffers, which causes great frustration among doctors and nurses, because most of them, if they don't have one, are specialising in Family Health, and are disappointed to find out what they should be doing and can't due to rules that don't comply with the Family Health Strategy. And the big problem is that the SES is not wrong, because the Ministry of Health gives autonomy to the states and municipalities to create their own regulations. The big problem is that the existing regulations predate the implementation of the strategy. Below are verbalisations that demonstrate the above:

> "We have to work with the team as public servants to provide the statistics that the secretariat requires of you, which are eminently **quantitative** statistics."
>
> **"It's often difficult to carry out** preventive work because **the professional is restricted to the consulting room."**
>
> **"There is also a demand that** the health department makes of the **professionals, which is 20 patients per period."**
> **"Quantity** is not a good service in our area of health. We deal with people, human beings. What's important to us is the **quality of** the service, the **care."**
>
> **"It's because they say 20, it's because 15 minutes per patient. That's 20 in five hours of** service, you know? So the PSF doesn't work like that. It's not about time, it's not about quantity, it's about **quality, the reason, the follow-up."**
>
> **"Quality is certainly** affected, for example, how are you going to be able to talk, get the patient to open up and everything in a **15-minute** consultation?"

The updated regulations that the SES/DF has published only refer to clinical conduct at all stages of life, covering all the programmes recommended by the Ministry. At this point in the Federal District there is not much to complain about, as there are good guidelines for clinical conduct. There may be a few flaws, but they are

The information provided in these publications, to which all professionals working in primary care have access, is few and far between.

The professionals also report on the need to improve the use of information available in the situation room, which is little used by everyone, as the report shows:

> **"There would have to be a situation room not just for the centre but for each team.** I think the process of **decentralisation** enhances action through information and then allows you to recentralise it. So if you have decentralisation in your situation room, you know the profile of your area, you know the profile of the other team's area and the manager can put this together. So I don't think it would have to be a single room for the centre, it would have to be a room for each team. (...) I don't think this kind of service should be delegated to a health professional, but to an administrative professional. The health professional whose knowledge could be used for something else, such as care and more meetings, for example. But the part of simply retrieving information that the system should give us is already done and doesn't cause these problems in the system. This would **be a huge** improvement for us."

5.1.4. Teamwork in the development of care actions

One of the main pillars of the PSF is teamwork, as different professionals work together to provide better solutions to patient needs.

Working in teams with population adscription seeks to overcome the past model, where most decisions and strategies were made by the doctor, who most of the time only provided care within the health unit and for an unknown clientele, making it difficult to maintain continuity of health actions. Now, these strategies are drawn up based on knowledge of the structure and real needs of the community, further emphasising the importance of the community health agent, who comes from that region and acts as an identifier of the problems that exist there. Furthermore, these problems can also be recognised by other members of the team, in the UBS itself or even in the community through home visits.

Once the problem has been identified, the team meets and analyses the material, technological and human resources available to solve it. A joint plan is then drawn up to define the intervention strategies that can be implemented with these resources. This allows the UBS to adapt to the needs of the community through flexible planning, unlike what happened in the past.

Therefore, the "team members articulate their practices and knowledge to tackle each situation identified in order to jointly propose solutions and intervene **appropriately, since everyone is familiar with the problem."(3)**

The response of one of the interviewees reflects this idea of looking to the group to solve problems:

> **"Teamwork** [is a positive point], because what we can't resolve we pass on to the group and we interact. Not just with our group, but there's the nutritionist, the social service, the dentist. The role of the ACS who bring the problems to us, because they're on the street and know the **reality better than we do."**

Since the teams are multi-professional and work from a multidisciplinary perspective, the professionals are able to assist and understand the patient as a whole. The patient is analysed as an individual who suffers bio-psycho-social influences according to the community in which they live and the people with whom they live. This approach is in line with the Operational Guidelines for the Family Health Programme, which proposes comprehensive care, **understood as "an articulated and continuous set of preventive and curative, individual and collective actions and services" (Law Number 8.080).**

5.1.5. Influence of personal motivation on the functioning of the Centre and personal opinions about the ESF

Some professionals don't believe that the conversion was a change to the family health strategy model. Some staff say that even with the conversion, the Health Centre is still not a PSF, because, as has already been said, this unit with several teams has characteristics that make it different from a unit with just one team. Among these differences we can mention the procedure rooms, such as vaccination, dressings and medication, which are unique to the three teams, and for this it is necessary to provide a nursing professional for each room, taking them away from the teams, which ends up creating various conflicts between the professionals and even a feeling of exclusion for those who are assigned to these rooms. According to the managers, there have already been attempts to rotate the nursing technicians between the teams in the rooms, but there were also conflicts, mainly because at the time of these attempts there were few nursing professionals, which made it very difficult to carry out all the activities planned for Family Health, such as home visits by this category, and it wasn't possible to schedule technicians in all the procedure rooms and in the teams' triage rooms.

However, with the arrival of more technicians at the unit, this changed and it was possible to restructure and put one technician in each room and three or four in each team.

Another difference is the fact that there is only one consulting room for each team, for the doctor and nurse to share, which is possible due to the daily working hours practised in all the basic units in the Federal District, which are 10 hours a day and not eight as is the case in most units in other states and even here in the Federal District in units that only have one team. This issue of working hours is a difference that influences the functioning of the activities recommended for the teams, since with one less day of work, the holding of ongoing team education and case discussion meetings is compromised.

The challenge for the SUS is to put together strategies that can effectively break with the current model of care. This is not for lack of trying. The large number of works produced in the area is proof of the attempts to change in the history of Brazilian public health. The PSF has emerged as a possible strategy for restructuring the SUS care model, with a view to overcoming this problem.

The following is a verbalisation that characterises the above.

> **"We're neither a centre nor a PSF**. Because I worked for many years as a family doctor in a little post office that used to be a PSF. So for me, this isn't a **PSF. But it's not a centre either, so...?"**

5.1.6. Relationship between physical structure, staff and demand

Organised teamwork and the logic of care divided into visits, procedures, consultations with a general practitioner and referrals, makes it more efficient to resolve complaints and there is an apparent view that there are more professionals involved in the family health strategy, as the following statement shows:

> "What's changed is that now there are **more doctors and more nurses."**

> **"...there are doctors, there are nurses, there are community workers, it's... even though they** are overloaded, the **team is complete so far."**

The problem therefore lies in the number of teams. Following the logic described above and considering the population served of almost 24,000 inhabitants, the health centre is serving twice its recommended capacity. This problem began with the appearance of the new settlement blocks, which represent more demand. As the following statement shows:

> **"We don'***t have* **a 100 per cent coverage area. There's a new** settlement **area** that doesn't have its own teams, these areas ended up being distributed among the teams that already exist. So today the population of out-of-area patients and patients in the team's area is almost the same. So the team that had to cater for a certain population is catering for twice as many."

We can clearly see that there was adequate demand at the start of the conversion, but new areas have sprung up and been distributed among the existing teams, when the right thing to do would have been to create new teams, just as they created new courts. New courts have sprung up without assistance, and this has even jeopardised the one that was well assisted.

> **"the reinforcement of** local **teams,** the sending of new doctors, the composition of new teams so that we can steer the ship more smoothly."

As already mentioned in the body of this paper, Ordinance 648/GM recommends that each team should serve an average of 3,000 people, up to a maximum of 4,000, and have enough CHWs to cover 100% of the registered population, with a maximum of 750 people per CHW, up to 12 CHWs per team(2). Any change in this ratio is detrimental to care and carrying out the activities recommended for the ESF - educational and care, individual and collective, home-based and intersectoral - requires a reduction in the number of families enrolled per ESF, and the recommendation of enrolling up to 1,000 families per ESF was considered too high to guarantee care for the population. This wide variation can be seen in the increase in the number of CHAs per team, which is reflected in the overload of higher education professionals. [4]

Another factor that has been identified as contributing to the increase in demand at this health unit is its good work, which attracts people from other places, relatives of people from the area and people who move away and continue to want to be seen. Some studies have pointed out that the change in the work process itself leads to an increase in spontaneous demand, which happens with the implementation of programmes that have the ACS facilitating the link with the community, whether PACS or ESF. [18]

> **"Because the** centre is so good, people come from **other places** to want to be seen **here."**

> **"There are cases of patients who move but continue to** use the same address to continue being seen here. There's also the case of relatives of patients from the centre who come to spend their **holidays and (...) use the card as if they were from here."**

Even so, due to the high demand, many residents complain about the service provided at the unit, especially when it comes to booking medical appointments. Some professionals say this is due to the curative mentality the population has.

In a study carried out in ten large urban centres in Brazil, the three main health problems mentioned by families enrolled in the PSF in eight of these urban centres were diseases, which were mentioned by all the municipalities. In second place in a greater number of municipalities, families mentioned problems with access to care and, lastly, aspects related to health professionals were reported, such as complaints about a lack of specialist doctors, a lack of professionals in care, a lack of dentists, a lack of home visits by doctors, difficulties for doctors in making diagnoses and a low number of home visits by CHAs. [26]

The family health strategy proposal also raises other needs that go beyond spontaneous demand, a silent demand that is identified by the welcoming attitude of the team[18] . To this end, health professionals have observed that other activities are hampered by the high demand, including the care of the low-risk population, the incorporation of health promotion actions and the care of highly complex cases, such as the reception and management of adolescent drug users.

> **"You can only get an appointment** if you're hypertensive, diabetic, pregnant or a child up to 2 years old. If you're older than 2, you can't."

"Here we don't have the structure to cater for young drug addicts, nor where to send them for treatment."

Thus, the teams have been facing the challenge of providing quality and resolutive care to all types of demand that come to the health unit, even with scarce resources.

Another limitation is the physical space. The conversion situation found at CSSam 03 uses the space of the traditional health centre to house some ESF teams. Bringing several teams together in the same place depends on administrative support, cleaning and security, as these activities support the work of the ESFs and make it possible for them to exchange information.

of staff, sharing of collective materials and support between one team and another, in these areas the conversion of the health centre structure was beneficial. [26]

This combination of teams is not a problem as long as there is an adequate physical area for each team: a doctor's and nurse's office for the team, a reception area/room, a place for files and records, a room for basic nursing care, a vaccination room and toilets, as well as adequate equipment and materials for the list of planned actions to ensure that the care provided is effective. The administration, test collection, pharmacy and immunisation departments can share resources. [4,26]

Ordinance 648/2006 MS recommends that each basic unit should have one to three teams, i.e. serve up to 12,000 inhabitants. If there is a need for a larger number of ESFs for the area, they should be located in basic units adjacent to the health centre or close to its catchment area, peripherally.

This combination can be understood as creating two levels of complexity within primary care. The teams are directly linked to the basic clinical specialities, increasing the resolution of complaints and making inter-consultation possible. [26]

5.1.7. Continuing education

For teamwork to work satisfactorily, each member needs to be aware of their duties and have the specific skills to fulfil them. To this end, in 2004 the Ministry of Health instituted the National Policy for Permanent Education in Health, which establishes human and **financial** resources for the **"training and development of health professionals, with a view to** strengthening the decentralisation of sector management, developing strategies and processes to achieve comprehensive individual and collective health care and increasing society's participation in the political decisions of the Unified Health System". **(17)**

However, it was clear from the interviews that continuing education for health professionals in Samambaia's Centro 3 is scarce, since there are no educational programmes at local level, which would be ideal, since each region has its own epidemiological characteristics and each UBS has different resources. There are only training programmes run by the Health Department (FEPECS) at district level. One interviewee made this shortcoming very clear:

> "There's no set schedule or frequency [of meetings]. They're actually meetings, even one-off meetings where we talk about a few things, but it doesn't really come down to an educational theme of running a class or doing further training. That's up to the health department itself. But there is an intention on the part of the team to carry out continuing education. We want to prepare these professionals in emergency care so that they can facilitate the care provided by doctors and nurses. What education there is for professionals is provided by the health department itself in one-off programmes and when there are events for CHAs to improve and educate them and workshops for doctors, nurses and nursing technicians."

Da Silva justifies the need to implement Continuing Health Education as follows:

> According to the Pan American Health Organisation (PAHO, 1978 apud Oguisso, 2000), continuing education is a dynamic, active and permanent teaching-learning process designed to update and improve the training of people or groups in the face of scientific and technological developments, social needs and institutional objectives and goals. Continuing education therefore needs to be considered as part of a global policy for the qualification of health workers, centred on the need to transform practice.

The proposal of the National Policy for Permanent Education in Health encompasses various changes in the activities and attitudes of health professionals, as well as in the logistics of the service and the physical structure of the health unit. To this end, the Ministry of Health has established five specific fields with objectives to be achieved:

- transforming the entire management and service network into school environments;

- to establish changes in training and health practices as a way of building comprehensive health care for the population;

- institute continuing education for SUS workers;

- building training and development policies on a local-regional basis;

- evaluation as a strategy for building an institutional commitment to co-operation and sustaining the process of change.

Continuing education takes place mainly in the UBS, in the form of **teaching and learning** activities. **In other words, in this context "Permanent Education is learning at** work, where learning and teaching are incorporated into the daily life of organisations and **work", according to the Ministry of Health. It is also proposed that the training of health professionals should be based on the "health needs of people and populations,** sector management and social control in health, have as their objectives the transformation of professional practices and the organisation of work itself and be structured based on the problematisation of the **work process."** [17]

5.2. Participant Observation

5.2.1. Doctor's observation

5.2.1.1. Knowledge of the Referral and Counter-referral System.

It was noted that professionals at the unit are fully aware of the referral and counter-referral system, but that it is poorly implemented because there are referrals but no counter-referrals. This is because the service's doctors refer users to medium and high-complexity services when necessary, but due to the lack of computerisation of the entire health network and the shortage of specialists in the network, it takes a long time for care to take place and when patients are seen, the patient's medical records don't always come back (counter-referral) and monitoring of the user's therapeutic plan, proposed by the referral and counter-referral, is hampered. (Brasil, 2006)

5.2.1.2. Carrying out basic health and epidemiological surveillance actions

They partially carry out basic health and epidemiological surveillance actions. The professional who sees a suspected case makes the Compulsory Notification, but the epidemiological investigation and control of compulsorily notifiable diseases and other diseases and situations of importance are carried out by a single nurse at the Health Centre who is responsible for the Health and Epidemiological Surveillance of all the teams and the entire region and population served by the Health Centre.

5.2.1.3. Carrying out consultations, diagnosis and treatment of individuals and families

They carry out diagnostic consultations and treatment of individuals and families.

> **"...in the PSF there's the** prenatal care **programme, the** CD **programme, the** group **programme, you** know, group meetings, pregnant women's meetings, CD meetings, visits, you know, and we **don't have that many opportunities for that."**

However, the requirement for consultations per shift is 20 patients, which means that comprehensive patient care is compromised.

> **"Certainly, the quality is affected, for example, how are you going to manage, is to talk, the patient opens up and everything in a 15-minute consultation."**

"The PSF doesn't work properly because of the demand and the demands...."

"**And** because they say 20, it's 15 minutes per patient. That's 20 in five hours of service, you see. So the PSF doesn't work like that. It's not about, it's not about, it's about, it's about **time, it's not about quantity, it's about quality, the reason, the follow-up.**"

5.2.1.4. Participation in team training, capacity building and continuing education.

It was noted that doctors do not take part in team training and continuing education. They report that due to high demand and other services, there is no time for planning or training and continuing education.

"**It weakens us a bit because we don't have meetings, because in a PSF we had** to have meetings every week. And we have one meeting a month and sometimes **no meeting at all.**"

"**And, because, there had** to be a meeting because there's no way that the ACS, me in the middle of the consultation, the ACS can talk about the problem. So it should be discussed in a meeting where we raise all the problems and things that could be resolved for the future. And as the aim here is consultation, consultation, consultation, you don't see this **part, so we end up not having it. So that's what I feel has been done.**"

Another point to be analysed is that according to ORDINANCE No. 648/GM OF 28th MARCH 2006.

"**In the Federal District, its Secretariat of** Health-SES is responsible for organising **the introductory course and/or the courses for the permanent education of the teams.**"

Therefore, continuing education is not the sole responsibility of doctors, but also of the SHS-DF

5.2.1.5. Planning and carrying out educational activities

It was noted that once a month the doctors, together with the nurse and CHAs from their team, hold meetings at the Health Centre for Diabetic and Hypertensive Groups. At these meetings there are talks about the disease in language that is very accessible to the patients and guidance on the importance of diet, physical activity and medication for the patients' well-being. After the meeting, all the patients in the group are seen by the doctor.

"**...the obligations that we have to keep more inside than** outside. Because the **meetings would ideally be held in the community, not here at the centre. But that's it.**" MD1

5.1.7.1. Filling in the Activity Production Register

They do. Because the activity production record is a control mechanism in which the Ministry of

Health verifies that the PSF is taking place and is therefore a way of evaluating the PSF. The Ministry of Health passes the buck to the PSF programme when it sees the activity production record.

5.1.7.2. Home visits

They do it partially, because they claim that due to the high demand for consultations at the Health Centre and the fact that consultations at the Centre are a priority, there is no time to carry out the weekly visits recommended by the PSF.

> **"And since the intention here is consultation, consultation, consultation, consultation..."**

They also claim that the Health Centre has to have at least one doctor, so if it's a visiting day but there's no other doctor at the Health Centre, the doctor stops making his visits and stays at the Health Centre to attend appointments.

> **"There are many times when _we_ can't leave** because there's only one doctor, we **can't go out for a visit."**

Visits are not made once a year to each family home, as recommended by the PSF (Ministry of Health, 2006). They are carried out according to need and risk situations that the CHA informs the team about.

5.2.2. Nurse observation

5.2.2.1. Monitoring the registration and updating of CHA data

This task is carried out, but not completely. The CHAs register and update the patients in the primary care information system (SIAB). At the end of the month, the nurse from each team checks all the data on paper and consolidates it to send to the central level. After this, an employee from GAPESF (Primary Care and Family Health Strategy Management) goes to the Health Centre, copies the data put into the system from all the teams and enters the data already checked into the programme at the regional level so that it can then be sent to the central level. This whole consolidation process is necessary because the SIAB is not an online system, but an MS-DOS system, used by the Ministry of Health for years without any updates. As a result, there ends up being two jobs, on paper and in the system, which results in poor and low utilisation of the SIAB for its true purpose, which is to use the data to propose improvement actions and team adjustments.

Although it is an activity carried out by the team nurse, there was no mention of it during the interview. This may be due to the nurses' lack of information about their duties, as recommended by the Ministry of Health through decree 648, or even because they underestimate the importance of this practice of supervising the work of CHAs, compared to their other duties.

5.2.2.2. Carrying out basic health and epidemiological surveillance actions

They promote health surveillance by supervising the recall of users with health problems, according to the health need identified (such as malnourished children, those with poor development, those who have missed a <u>vaccination</u>). (PERES, 2006)

It was noted that this function is partially carried out because there is a specific surveillance professional in the unit who does most of the work, specifically the bureaucratic work. The nurse makes notifications and also coordinates the active search actions carried out by the auxiliaries and CHAs in her area of coverage, evaluates and monitors cases of tuberculosis and leprosy, in a context of mutual help, since there is also a professional assigned to monitor these cases who is a nurse who only works at the unit for 20 hours and cannot take on any team due to her workload. Notifications are the responsibility of the professional (doctor and nurse) who attended to the case. During the interviews, the above fact was confirmed, as shown in the speech below:

> "I do epidemiological surveillance, it's something the teams should do, but it's the unit that does it."

The nurse's partial performance of this activity is backed up by the fact that the health centre model is different from the PSF team standardised by the Ministry of Health. The health centre already had a support service for epidemiological surveillance activities, which is characterised by the existence of its own person to carry out the investigation and control. This makes it easier to keep track of all the cases, so as not to miss any surveillance action, which has deadlines for being carried out, as there is a high demand for activities for the team nurse.

5.2.2.3. Planning, execution and coordination and helping to organise the basic health unit

This activity consists of planning and evaluating nursing activities; delegating and distributing tasks to staff; supervising the nursing team and the activities carried out; being responsible for forecasting and providing the material and equipment needed for nursing activities; helping to maintain appliances and equipment and, when necessary, requesting repairs; drawing up and updating nursing procedures, routines and standards; periodically reviewing data records and communication systems; analysing and evaluating the care provided to the community. (PERES, 2006)

The nurse carries out this activity, since he is responsible for supervising and coordinating the nursing assistants and CHAs in his team. Some professionals mentioned this activity during the interviews.

The only thing the nurse doesn't do is stock up on materials and equipment; he anticipates, but doesn't order, because due to the computerisation of the entire Health Centre, there is a computerised system for this purpose and there is also a server responsible for carrying out these orders. All the other actions are carried out by the nurse, which demonstrates the great overload of activity under the nurse's responsibility and shows how difficult it is for them to reach the target of daily consultations required by the SES/DF, through its Manual of Norms and Parameters, which, being out of date, was not written taking into account all these actions of the ESF.

5.2.2.4. Monitoring and evaluation of nursing care for individuals and their families

It consists of comprehensive care for individuals and families at the USF and, when indicated or necessary, at home and/or in other community spaces, at all stages of human development. In accordance with the protocols and other technical regulations established by the district manager, and in compliance with the legal provisions of the profession, they carry out nursing consultations. (FERRAZ, 2007)

It's the activity most often carried out, since there is a certain priority for this function and even personal satisfaction for the professionals who do it. Almost all the nurses mentioned this activity during the interviews, and their practice was also observed. Only the head nurse, who is responsible for administration and coordinating the services of all the teams, is exempt from this role.

With the conversion, nursing activities, especially consultations, were the main difference between the Health Centre before and after the conversion. Nurses' work was valued. Patients have learnt to respect and enjoy their work. And this brings a lot of satisfaction to these professionals, who have all their knowledge and skills utilised to the full, enabling a significant increase in patient access to the unit to have their needs met.

The nurse organises his monthly activities, which cover all the basic programmes recommended by the Ministry of Health, through a monthly schedule of activities that he leaves in the teams' triage room, so that everyone can know what kind of care will be provided each day of the month. This timetable also includes time off and time away from the unit so that patients are not surprised by any cancellations.

As well as organising, he often reviews his approaches to patients, such as educational meetings, home visits and even dressings, in order to improve care.

5.2.2.5.   Promoting training and continuing education for the nursing team

The educational functions are related to the training of the nursing team, where she identifies the needs of the staff, plans, executes and evaluates the courses given. Promotes educational activities with users during consultations, during home visits and in group work, with a view to individual autonomy in relation to health prevention, promotion and rehabilitation. Discusses health problems and alternatives for resolving them with organised groups in society (landless groups, residents' associations, churches and others) (PERES, 2006).

This activity is not carried out consistently. It was observed that educational activities for the nursing team are carried out sporadically and based on the current needs of the service. Sporadic training is not given individually to each team, but one person from the health centre is responsible for preparing lectures, which must be presented to all the teams.

There was a lack of responsibility on the part of the nurse or local management to coordinate such actions. The difficulty encountered by nursing professionals in carrying out educational activities for the team is the lack of time, since there are prioritisation criteria, and this is considered to be an action of less relevance to the functioning of the service. The professionals report that it is recommended that a weekly and a monthly meeting be held between the team's professionals to discuss the problems of the patients being cared for and thus promote education through experiential reality, but the opening hours of the health centre in the Federal District, which are 10 hours a day, make this practice impossible.

The Federal District assumes responsibility for training team professionals through FEPECS - the Foundation for Teaching and Research in Health Sciences, an organ of the SES/DF responsible for all SES/DF training. However, these are always geared more towards higher education professionals and less towards mid-level professionals. In addition, the difficulty of releasing all the professionals to take the courses was mentioned, and it often happens that there is more than one course at the same time.

5.2.2.6.   Home visits

It is an instrument in the set of tools (techniques, procedures and knowledge) of collective health nursing, used to intervene in the family health-disease process, carried out at the place of residence, rather than at the place of work or study. As an area of activity, it is one of nursing's own activities, in a broad approach that aims to extend health actions to the population, within a social context. (EGRY, 2000)

Visits are carried out based on the needs reported by the CHAs and are not organised in such a way as to cover the entire population covered by the team. The Ministry of Health recommends that every family should be visited at least once a year by the nurse. This is not done due to the high demand for other services, which leaves home visits as the last task to be carried out. Although each team's diary contains times set aside for home visits, it was observed that these times were almost always used for other activities.

During the interviews, this activity was mentioned by only one nurse, which demonstrates the low level of practice of this function in this professional category. This was also confirmed during participant observation, where no home visits were seen by nurses.

5.2.3. Observation by Community Health Agents

Considering the context and conceptions of health that have the Brazilian Health Reform as a doctrinal reference and the Single Health System as a strategy for sectoral and institutional reorganisation, the professional competence of health workers is understood as one of the fundamental components for the desired qualitative revolution in health services (BRASIL, 2003).

CHWs work to support individuals and social groups, identifying the most common health risk situations, participating in guidance, monitoring and popular health education, extending the responsibilities of local health teams, putting into action knowledge about the prevention and solution of health problems, mobilising practices to promote collective life and the development of social interactions.

5.2.3.1.   Monthly monitoring of all the families under their responsibility, through home visits.

Home visits are one of the main activities recommended by the Ministry of Health for community health workers (Brasil, 2001) and were also the most mentioned in this study. It is recommended to encourage regular monthly home visits by CHWs, which requires reducing the number of families per ESF.

> "Home visits, attending lectures and booking people in. Checking patients' medication."
>
> "I make home visits".

The agent is responsible for 750 people in their community, and this number is flexible as it depends on local needs. They must visit each household at least once a month (FERRAZ, 2005). However, for most agents, it is not possible to visit every family every month, as the number is too high. This situation was evident in this study, which means that, according to the agents interviewed, they have to prioritise the families that need more monitoring. It is recommended to encourage regular monthly home visits by CHWs, which requires a reduction in the number of families per ESF. (BRASIL, 2005) Another problem mentioned by CHWs for not carrying out monthly visits is the fact that many families work and no member of the family is left at home during the CHWs' visiting hours. It's clear then that only home-based enrolment makes it difficult for workers to receive care, and it's advisable to study the possibility of registering by place of work, through individual enrolment at USFs close to the place of work. We can also encourage USFs to open at times that allow workers to access them (BRASIL, 2005).

5.2.3.2. Strengthening the link between individuals/families/community and the health service

According to the Ministry of Health, the CHW is a worker who is part of the health team in the community where they live, and their main task is to establish a link between these two universes.

Some CHWs interviewed emphasised this role.

"My job is to provide a link between the community and the health centre."

It was observed that without the CHAs, the creation of bonds, which many professionals emphasise as a positive point in the PSF, would not be possible. They fulfil this function satisfactorily since, being part of the community, they know its problems and so can bring them to the team in search of solutions.

5.2.3.3. Mapping your micro-area and registering families

When all CHWs join a PSF team, they are assigned to a specific micro-area, the population of which they are responsible for. The mapping of the area is done during the first home visits, where a demographic, social and pathological survey of each family is carried out. After this task, the CHWs enter the registered families into the health centre's system and update them when necessary. The nurse of each team monitors and coordinates the work of the CHWs.

This activity was also mentioned by some CHAs during the interviews.

"We have to update families and productivity in the system."

It was also noted during participant observation that all CHWs carried out this activity. The majority of CHAs interviewed did not report this activity. This can be attributed to the fact that this function is carried out when they first come into contact with the family, and is therefore not part of their daily routine.

5.2.3.4. Guidance for the community on the right to health and how to access it

In fact, the community has some knowledge of the link that the CHW makes with the health service. Thus, it was observed that the CHWs are often sought out by the population they assist to obtain information about the possibilities of appointments or services at the Health Centre. It is the CHW who brings the needs of the population to the team.

The CHWs register families and inform them which team they belong to. They also advise patients that if they need anything, they should go to their team at the health centre. In this way, the CHWs help organise the service by guiding patients.

5.2.4. Nursing Technician

5.2.4.1. Identifying families in situations of risk and monitoring
          their individuals together with the ACS

They don't. Families at risk are identified exclusively by the CHWs, who make home visits every day. The nursing technicians don't make routine visits. The CHA reports the risk situation and, depending on the need and situation, the technicians make the home visit accompanied by the CHA.

> **"It's the CHWs who choose, they prioritise,** who needs it most, because they always visit, right, they see who needs it most and they take us to **the houses."**

5.2.4.2. Cleaning, disinfecting, sterilising, conserving and
          storing equipment and service equipment.

It was noted that the assistant is responsible for organising, storing and conserving the materials and equipment used collectively by his team, such as thermometers, sphygmomanometers, scales, measuring tapes, blood glucose meters, anthropometers and stethoscopes. The materials that need to be disinfected and sterilised are the responsibility of the Health Centre's only nursing technician, who collects the used material and cleans, disinfects and sterilises it, as well as providing the material according to the needs of the Health Centre and the teams.

> **"I usually** stay here with the materials. I only stay in the teams when **there's a problem there."**

5.2.4.3. Nursing care and procedures at home

They do. The nursing assistants at the Health Centre are assigned to the Vaccination Room, the Medication Room and the Dressing Room. Although the assistants have their own specific teams, when they are in these rooms they meet all the demand at the Centre. What's more, the population doesn't have to wait for the nursing technician in their team to leave and attend to them. When they are assigned to the triage room, however, they only attend to their team, due to the high demand in the triage room.

> "I'm in the triage room, I'm also a trained employee in the vaccination room, we do dressings, medication, all the duties of a nursing technician, we do them here. "

5.2.3.5. Home visits

It was observed that the nursing technicians partially carry out home visits. There were no routine visits by the technicians, only sporadic visits to patients who had some priority such as bedridden, post-surgical, handicapped or at risk, as reported by the CHWs.

In interviews, the nursing technicians themselves recognised the importance of home visits and the failure to carry out this requirement.

> **"Normally, care has to be provided at home. But normally the** home visit is, it allows us to solve a range of problems in the community, instead of having this flow, a lot of people here at the Post, right, having this demand, which is very high. So, in the community we'd do much better."

They explain the high demand for patients at the health centre, the lack of time for home visits and personal dissatisfaction with home visits.

> "I really don't like it, to say I like it, I don't like it. If I said I liked it, I'd be lying. But I can see that it's very good, you know."

It was observed that nursing technicians, because they work at the front door, i.e. they are the professionals who receive all the patients who come to the Health Centre, their complaints and try to resolve them in the best possible way, are the most overloaded professionals during the period from 7:00 am to 10:00 am and the professionals who complain the most about the overload and report greater stress and have a higher rate of sick leave due to health problems.

> **"The entrance door** is now the triage of each team. So, from suckling to lactating, they'll enter through that door, if they want prevention, to resolve a fever, they'll go to that room and that's very good. And from that room, depending on the need, he'll be booked in, seen or referred to hospital depending on the situation, and he'll be **seen by the doctor in the area."** "We book appointments, return visits, triage patients so they can be referred to the doctor and give patients the information they need."

However, it was observed that after 10am these professionals are idle, a time when home visits could be carried out, a function that is partially carried out by these professionals who claim that they don't carry out visits due to the high demand at the Health Centre and because they don't like carrying them out.

> **"We do the triage, we make home visits when we can."**

> **"I don't visit, because I hate visiting. I've always** said that I don't like **visiting".**

> **"I'm a nursing technician. I triage patients and book** appointments (...) Occasionally I'm in the medication room (...) I also **do** dressings **and occasionally I make visits too."**

5.3. Comparison of reality with Ordinance 648/2006

To better visualise the assessment made by comparing the items

The table below identifies the items recommended by Ordinance 648/2006 MS with the reality observed in the health unit that is the object of this research, facilitating comparison. We then discuss the items in order to better understand them.

Items evaluated	Preconised by Ordinance 648	Observed reality
Territory and population	12,000 inhabitants / 3 ESF / 1 UBS	24,000 inhabitants / 3 ESF / 1 UBS
Human Resources	1 doctor 1 nurse 1 nursing assistant 4 to 6 CHWs	1 doctor 1 nurse 3 nursing technicians 3 ACS
Workload	8 hours a day 5 days a week 40 hours per week	10 hours a day 4 days a week 40 hours per week
Physical Structure	Medical practice Nurse's surgery Reception area/room Place for files and records Basic care room (medication and dressing) Vaccination room Toilets	Joint office for doctor and nurse for each team Gynaecology practice Specialist practice Nutrition Consultancy Multi-purpose office Team reception
	Equipment	Archive Medication room and care Dressing room Vaccination room Meeting room CHA room Pharmacy Administrative Rooms Cup Patient toilets Staff toilets Equipment ok
Reference and Contra Reference	There is an organised system	Referral exists and works, counter-referral is poor.
Permanent extra-team education	State responsibility	Accordingly, with reservations
Permanent intra-team education	-	Sporadic
Involvement of managers	Recommended responsibilities for each sphere of government	Undefined local responsibilities
Cover	100%	Around 35%*

*Taking into account the population registered in the SIAB up to December 2009.

5.3.1. Territory and population

Samambaia Health Centre No. 03 has a population that exceeds the recommended number of teams. Mapping shows that there are many unregistered families, even within the area covered by the teams, due to the insufficient number of Community Health Agents.

What's more, with the new settlement that was created a year and a half ago, the population has practically doubled and there has been no incentive, no prioritisation of professionals to work in this uncovered area. According to managers, even with insufficient physical space, it would be better to have more professionals to meet this demand than to continue as we are, with adequate physical space for three teams and demand that exceeds the possibility of offering a quality service.

Quality is completely compromised by the enormous demand, which also generates a great deal of stress for the professionals who see all the work that has been going on, especially in terms of disease prevention and health promotion, being interrupted. This frustrates everyone.

5.3.2. Human Resources

As far as human resources are concerned, the Federal District has a special feature, since the Federal District's State Health Department took over the programme, which is that it only hires through public tenders, which is not the case in most of Brazil's municipalities, which use employment contracts with town halls, or sometimes hold tenders to hire through the CLT. On the one hand, this is very good, as it reduces turnover, especially among higher education professionals. However, it also delays the relocation of professionals who leave.

At Health Centre No. 03, in terms of staff numbers, the number of Community Health Agents is insufficient even for the teams that are registered and considered complete, which have only 3 to 4 CHAs for each, requiring five. When we were finalising the data collection, the unit received 10 more CHAs, five to work in rural areas and five to be divided between the teams. However, there was no prioritisation of the settlement, which still has no team.

In addition to the need not only for CHAs, but also for at least three more teams, although the NASF is not the subject of our work, we realise that the professionals to work in it are scarce, with only one gynaecologist with 40 hours, a paediatrician with only 15 hours, and a nutritionist with 20 hours who is on maternity leave. There are no doctors, no social workers and no other professionals who would be important to support the NASF. This lack of enough teams to cater for the entire population has led to great dissatisfaction among the NASF professionals, who are no longer supporting the general practitioners, and end up only attending to external demand, in order to reduce user dissatisfaction due to the lack of doctors.

Dentistry is another problem in terms of being registered in the teams, because the unit has two dentists, but one only works 20 hours and the other works 30 hours, as she is the head of the regional dentistry department for 10 hours. It's not possible to register them in the teams.

5.3.3. Workload

The health centres in the Federal District have a 10-hour workday, so the professionals don't work five days a week but four, which ends up reducing some of the strategy's activities, such as weekly team meetings for continuing education, and extra-mural activities, i.e. outside the health centre, such as schools and other community institutions. These activities are carried out by the teams, but always to the detriment of others, the biggest detriment being the home visit, which because there is no appointment, i.e. the patient is not waiting, the time set aside for it is used to carry out other activities, including bureaucratic activities such as monthly productivity.

5.3.4. Physical Structure

The physical structure of Health Centre No. 03 is adequate for three teams, despite not having a doctor's office and a nurse's office for each team, but it is insufficient for the number of teams that the unit's catchment area needs.

In general, Health Centre No. 03 has a good physical structure, with well-distributed and well-lit rooms, but they are poorly ventilated, generating dissatisfaction among the staff. However, it has all the rooms required by the Ministry of Health: reception/screening rooms, consulting rooms, a filing cabinet, a pharmacy, a dressing room, a medication room, a vaccination room, a meeting room, a room for the CHAs, an administrative area, a test collection room, and separate toilets for patients and staff. It is also very clean, well-kept, tree-lined and has a car park for staff. It's a good unit compared to others in Samambaia itself. Of course, there's always room for improvement.

5.3.5. Referral and Counter-Referral

The professionals who work at the unit in question are familiar with how to refer patients to secondary and tertiary care, and because it is a previously structured health centre, this is a positive aspect of the conversion. Most of the family health units described in other works have a lot of difficulty in referring patients, but here this difficulty is less because there is a whole structured network of care.However, this does not mean that there are no problems. On the contrary, there are many, because the network is structured, but it doesn't have enough professionals at secondary and tertiary level to meet all the demand. As a result, patients spend a long time waiting to be called for an appointment with a specialist. The team's professionals also complain that counter-referrals don't happen. The patient goes and if he doesn't come back to say what happened, the team doctor doesn't know. To solve this problem, the Federal District has a courier system for sending patients' medical records when they are referred to another level, but most of the time this medical record is returned with minimal information, making it impossible to know how the patient was treated and cared for.

Another solution that has begun, also with Health Centre No. 03 as a reference, is the computerisation of the entire network. This is already working in Samambaia, but unfortunately it hasn't yet spread to the other regional centres. The computerisation of medical records in Samambaia was widely cited by civil servants as an excellent initiative, which also has problems, but which has made it possible to improve care.

5.3.6. Extra- and intra-team continuing education

It was realised that there is a lack of in-patient educational practices, which should be carried out by doctors and nurses. This is due to the limited time and high demand at the centre, making it impossible to set aside a day a week exclusively for such practices. These practices are extremely important, as they provide the necessary support to achieve a comprehensive service, and for team meetings and the development of strategies to have a scientific basis.

The Federal District also takes on the training of FHP professionals in all primary care programmes through FEPECS - the Foundation for Teaching and Research in Health Sciences. However, there are organisational problems that make it impossible to release staff to attend courses, such as concurrent courses, where it is impossible for professionals to attend two courses at the same time; courses for all professionals, where it is not possible for the Health Centre to close for professionals to attend courses, among other problems.

5.3.7. Managers' involvement in implementing the Family Health Strategy

It's clear from various literature that in order to successfully implement the family health strategy, managers at all levels need to be heavily involved. This was also felt here at Health Centre No. 03. In the beginning, managers were more involved in making the conversion a reality, although not as everyone would have liked, especially in terms of training. Then, with successive changes of management, the general feeling among staff is one of abandonment. Mainly because, after two years, various problems have arisen that require intervention by higher authorities, which is not happening.

Participatory and knowledgeable management is essential for converting a health centre.

CHAPTER 6

Final considerations

The initial proposal of the family health programme corresponds to the needs of the community and would be effective if applied to adequate demand and sufficient resources. We have seen this in the many positive results found in this research. However, there are still many changes that need to be made to the programme's standardisation and regulation of actions, as well as evaluating the effectiveness of this strategy. The operation of the converted health centre should be seen as something that differs from both the conventional centre and the family health programme, to function as a third, more complex structure. The existence of several teams in the same location has already been indicated in other studies as a good alternative for large urban centres and is not a problem as long as it has the right structure for the number of teams and a compatible population.

One interesting result of the conversion strategy was the greater interaction between the professionals who work in the teams, because before each one stayed in a room and there was no kind of team relationship. Today, the professionals from the same team work together and interact a lot with the staff from the other teams, because they always need mutual help, especially to fit patients in on days when a doctor from one of the teams is absent. However, it was also observed that there are intra- and extra-team conflicts, and in order to improve this situation, team meetings are held monthly at Samambaia's Centre 03. These meetings are extremely important because the problems encountered by the team are discussed and intervention strategies are developed jointly. This means that decisions are no longer centred on doctors, but on a multiprofessional and multidisciplinary approach, as well as the participation of the ACS, who knows the region and its needs. As a result, strategies become more specific and therefore more effective.

It was also noted that the centralisation of the Federal District government hampers the proper functioning of the unit, as the Regional Health Centre has no autonomy to solve certain problems, especially with regard to finances. If a tap breaks in the unit, it can't be fixed, because there are no resources to solve the problem, neither in the Regional Health Office, nor in the Health Centre.

The staff plan to hold a bazaar at least twice a year to raise money to buy small items that the unit needs, and even to make small repairs themselves.

Another point raised here, as in all of Brazil, is doctor turnover, since **according to CONASS (2007), "the figure of the doctor has been pointed out as a critical node** in the evolution of the ESF, due to its high turnover and, in some cases, little training for **PHC work".** This is also the case at Health Centre No. 03. However, contrary to the statistics, of the three teams, two have had the same doctors for more than three years, and both are specialists in Family and Community Health.

Finally, the conversion broadened the scope of professional activity, valuing the performance of nursing in primary care in particular. There was also an increase in the involvement of professionals with the population, reflecting a major contribution to resolving patient problems, but also in various demands on all levels of management to solve problems in the health system. Furthermore, the conversion was only successful due to the commitment, involvement and performance of all the professionals who took part in this process.

Recommendations

Converting a traditional health centre into a Family Health Strategy can be a great way to restructure primary care, provided that:

® There is prior training for the professionals who will work in the new model;

® Sufficient teams are offered to cover the unit's catchment area;

® Adequate physical space is made available, if not inside, then in areas adjacent to the unit.

® There is a local manager committed to the family health strategy and its operation.

® Involvement of all strategy managers, at regional and central level, in the whole process.

CHAPTER 7

Bibliographical references

1. GOULART, FLÁVIO A. DE ANDRADE. Experiences in Family Health: each case is different? Thesis (Doctorate in Public Health) - National School of Public Health, **Oswaldo Cruz Foundation**, Rio de Janeiro 2002, 387p. : il. Available at: http://www.bireme.br/php/index.php. Accessed on 20 July 2009.

2. BRAZIL. MINISTRY OF HEALTH. Practical Guide to the Family Health Programme, **Ministry of Health. Department of Primary Care.** 2001. 128p.

3. NEVES, C. F.; CAVALCANTE, J. P. R.; BEZERRA, J. I. A.; PEREIRA, J. F.; PITTERI, J. S. M.; BARBOSA, M. A. - **Perceptions of the population about the family health programme in Palmas-TO.** Revista da UFG, Vol. 6, No. Especial, Dec 2004, available at: www.proec.ufg.br Accessed on 10 May 2009

4. BRAZIL. Ministry of Health. Ordinance 648/ GM of 28 March 2006. Ministry of Health.   2006. Available at:
http://dtr2001.saude.gov.br/sas/PORTARIAS/Port2006/GM/GM-648.htm Accessed on: 15 March 2008

5. SILVEIRA C. H.; PINTO D. K. Oficinas de Planejamento Local em Saúde para o Programa de Saúde da família com enforque estratégico em Joinville-SC Revista Espaço para a Saúde, Londrina, v.1,   n.2, p. 196-204, jun. 2000. Available at:
http://www.ccs.uel.br/espacoparasaude/v1n2/relatos de experiencia1.htm Accessed on: 18 Nov 2009.

6. BRAZIL. Ministry of Health. Manual for the physical structure of basic health units : family health / Ministry of Health, Secretariat for Health Care, Department of Primary Care - 2. ed. - Brasília : Ministry of Health, 2008. 52 p. : il. colour - (Series A. Standards and Technical Manuals)

7. TESTA M. Pensamento estratégico e lógica de programação: o caso da Saúde. São Paulo: Hucitec; 1995.

8. MENDES EV. An agenda for Health. São Paulo: Hucitec; 1996.

9. PAIM JS. Health reform and care models. In: Rouquayrol MZ, organiser. Epidemiology and health. 5th ed. São Paulo: Hucitec; 1999. p. 473-87.

10. BRAZIL. Ministry of Health. Seminar on International Experiences in Family Health: report of a working group. Brasília: MS; 2000.

11. BRAZIL. National Council of Municipal Health Secretaries. Primary Care and Health Promotion/ . Brasília: CONASS, 2007. 232 p.

12. TRAD LAB, BASTOS ACS. The socio-cultural impact of the Family Health Programme (PSF): a proposal for evaluation. Cad Saúde Pública. Rio de Janeiro, v. 14, n. 2, Apr. 1998. Available at <http://www.scielo.br/scielo.php?script=sci_arttext&pid=S0102- 311X1998000200028&lng=en&nrm=iso>. accessed on 29 Apr. 2010. doi: 10.1590/S0102- 311X1998000200028. Accessed on 18 July 2009.

13. **LEUCOVITZ, E.; GARRIDO, N.G.** Saúde da Família: a procura de um modelo **anunciado**. Cadernos de Saúde da Família, ano I, n°1, jan. - jun. 1996, p.3-9.

14. TEIXEIRA, M. B. Empowerment of the elderly in groups aimed at health promotion. [Master's Degree] Oswaldo Cruz Foundation, National School of Public Health; 2002. 105 p. Chapter 4 , available at : http://portalteses.icict.fiocruz.br/transf.php?script=thes chap&id=00003404&lng=en&n rm=isso, Accessed 01 Aug 2009.

15. BRASIL. Constituição da República Federativa do Brasil: texto constitucional promulgado em 5 de outubro de 1988, Brasília, Senado Federal, Subsecretaria de edições Técnicas, 2002. 72 p.

16. HUBNER, Luiz Carlos Moreira; FRANCO, Túlio Batista. The family doctor programme in Niterói as a strategy for implementing a model of care that takes into account the principles and guidelines of the SUS. Physis , Rio de Janeiro, v. 17, n. 1, 2007 . Available at:

<http://www.scielo.br/scielo.php?script=sci_arttext&pid=S0103- 73312007000100010&lng=pt&nrm=iso>. Accessed on: 04 Aug 2009

17. BRAZIL. Ministry of Health. Secretariat for Labour Management and Health Education. Department of Health Education Management.Política Nacional de Educação Permanente em Saúde / Ministry of Health, Secretariat of Labour Management send Health Education, Department of Health Education Management. - Brasília : Ministry of Health, 2009. 64 p. - (Series B. Textos Básicos de Saúde) (Series Pactos pela Saúde

2006; v. 9)

18.	SILVA, Teresa Cristina Santos A construção das práticas de integralidade no cotidiano de uma equipe de saúde da família/Teresa Cristina Santos Silva. BeloHorizonte, 2006149f. Available at: http://www.enf.ufmg.br/mestrado/dissertacoes/TeresaCristina.pdf Accessed on: 05 August 2009

19.	HUBNER, Luiz Carlos Moreira; FRANCO, Túlio Batista. The family doctor programme in Niterói as a strategy for implementing a model of care that takes into account the principles and guidelines of the SUS. **Physis** , Rio de Janeiro, v. 17, n. 1, 2007 . Available at: <http://www.scielo.br/scielo.php?script=sci_arttext&pid=S0103-73312007000100010&lng=pt&nrm=iso>. Accessed on: 04 Aug 2009.

20.	VALENTIM, M. Métodos de Pesquisa: Análise de Conteúdo Department of Information Science, Universidade Estadual Paulista/ Faculdade de Filosofia e Ciências, Marília, 2008.

21.	MINAYO, M. C. S. **O Desafio do Conhecimento - Pesquisa Qualitativa em Saúde.** São Paulo: Hucitec/Rio de Janeiro: Abrasco, 1992. 269 p

22.	BONI V.; QUARESMA S. J. **Aprendendo a entrevistar: como fazer entrevistas em Ciências Sociais.** Revista Eletrônica dos Pós-Graduação em Sociologia Política da UFSC Vol. 2 n° 1 (3), January-July/2005, p. 68-80.

23.	QUEIROZ D. T.; VALL J.; SOUZA, A. M. A.; VIEIRA, N. F. C. **Participant observation in qualitative research: concepts and applications in the health area.** Rev. enferm. UERJ v.15 n.2 Rio de Janeiro April/June 2007.

24.	CHIZZOTTI A. **Research in the humanities and social sciences.** Cortez, São Paulo, 1995.

25.	BRAZIL, Ministry of Health. **Evaluation for Improving the Quality of the Family Health Strategy - technical document.** Secretariat of Health Care, Department of Primary Care, Brasília, Ministry of Health, 2005. Series B. Basic Health Texts.

26.	ROSA, Walisete de Almeida Godinho; LABATE, Renata Curi. Family health programme: building a new model of care. Rev. Latino-Am. Enfermagem , Ribeirão Preto, v. 13, n. 6, 2005 . Available at: http://www.scielo.br/scielo.php?script=sci arttext&pid=S0104-11692005000600016&lng=en&nrm=iso

Accessed: 04 Aug 2009

27.   ESCOREL, Sarah et al. Saúde da Família: avaliação da implementação em dez grandes centros urbanos: síntese dos principais resultados / Ministério da Saúde, Fundação Oswaldo Cruz; 2. ed. atual. - Brasília: Ministry of Health Publishing House, 2005. 210 p.: ill. Available in   : http://dab.saude.gov.br/docs/geral/avaliacao psf sintese grandescentros.pdf Accessed on: 06 August 2009.

28.   **AGUIAR José Manuel Monteiro d'.** The Family Health Programme in Brazil. A resolutividade do PSF no município de Volta Redonda (RJ) ENSP/FIOCRUZ Rio de Janeiro, 2001,   147p.
        Disponívelem   :   http://bases.bireme.br/cgi-bin/wxislind.exe/iah/online/?IsisScript=iah/iah.xis&src=google&base=LILACS&lang=p&nextAction=lnk&exprSearch=284164&indexSearch=ID Accessed: 06 Aug 2009

29.   **AGUIAR, Dayse Santos. Family Health in the Unified Health System: A** New Paradigm? Oswaldo Cruz Foundation. National School of Public Health. Rio de Janeiro, 1998,175p. Available at: http ://bases.bireme.br/cgi-bin/wxislind.exe/iah/online/?IsisScript=iah/iah.xis&src=google&base=LILACS&lang=p&nextAction=lnk&exprSearch=232415&indexSearch=ID Accessed on 06 Aug 2009.

30.   ARAÚJO, Mariza Sandra de Souza. Água Mole em Pedra Dura?Organisational changes in the Rio Grande do Norte Public Health Department following the implementation of the new system.

of the Family Health Programme. Ministry of Health. Oswaldo Cruz Foundation. Aggeu Magalhães Research Centre. Department of Collective Health/Nesc. Recife, 2000, 152p.

CHAPTER 8

ANNEXES

INFORMED CONSENT FORM

1. You are being invited to take part as a volunteer in the research: "Evaluation of the functioning of a traditional Health Centre converted into a Family Health Strategy in the Federal District" involving the staff of the Family Health teams at Samambaia Health Centre No. 03. It consists of answering a questionnaire with open questions about the functioning of the Family Health Strategy in this unit. The interview will be carried out individually with each participant by a medical student from the School of Health Sciences who is a member of the research group.

2. The aim of the study was to assess the relationship between the existing organisational structure of the health centre and that recommended by the Ministry of Health.

3. You will receive all the information and have your questions answered. There will be no discomfort, cost or risk.

4. You are free not to take part and you can withdraw at any stage and there will be no harm to you in doing so. You are free to refuse to answer any question in this questionnaire.
The results of the research will be publicised at GAPESF and throughout the Samambaia Regional Hospital, and may even be published at a later date. The data and materials used in the research will be kept by the Health Unit carrying out the project.

5. The data collected will be exclusively for the proposed research project, the information obtained will be confidential and the results of the study will be available for your knowledge. The results obtained in this study will be disseminated at the Health Centre, the Samambaia Regional Hospital and the School of Health Sciences No. 03 and may be used for presentations at congresses and medical journals. Once published, they will not contain personal information and will be stored on computer for five (5) years.

6. This form will be available in two copies, for the interviewee and the researcher, and the researchers will be available for any clarification.
Researchers responsible and contact telephone numbers:
Enf Charmene de Alcântara Marques Menezes (Supervisor): (61) 8428-4678

Aline Nunes Batista: (61) 9842-8811

Nubia Kátia Teixeira dos Santos: (61) 9618-6654

SES/DF Research Ethics Committee: 3325 4955.

7. Have you decided to take part in this study? Signing this consent form means that you have decided to volunteer after reading and understanding all the information provided and contained in this form.

Brasilia, _____ 2009.

Name of participant:

ID:_____________________ Signature: ____

Name and signature of the researcher: ____

Annex II

QUETIONARY

Semi-structured interview with professionals from the Samambaia Health Centre No. 03:

1. What are your functions within this unit?
2. What changes have you seen in the operation of CSSam 03 with the conversion?
3. What positive points would you highlight as the most important in the operation of Samambaia Health Centre No. 03? (Name 03)
4. What negative points would you highlight as the most relevant in the operation of Samambaia Health Centre No. 03? (Name 03)

Annex III

Script for observing the functional reality of Health Centre No. 03 in Samambaia.

Items to look out for	R	PR	N R	Observations
Knowledge of the referral and counter-referral system;				
Carrying out basic health and epidemiological surveillance actions;				
Carrying out consultations, diagnosis and				

M É D I C O	treatment of individuals and families;				
	Participation in the process of training, capacity building and continuing education for the teams;				
	Planning and carrying out educational activities;				
	Filling in the activity production log;				
	Home visits.				
E N F E R M E I R A	Monitoring of registration and updating of data by CHAs;				
	Helping to organise the basic health unit;				
	Carrying out basic health and epidemiological surveillance actions;				
	Planning, execution, coordination, Monitoring and evaluation of nursing care for individuals and their families;				
	Promoting training and continuing education for the nursing team;				
	Home visits.				
T IS C. E N F.	Identifying families in situations of risk and monitoring their individuals together with the CHWs;				
	Cleaning, disinfection, sterilisation, conservation and storage of the service's material and equipment;				
	Nursing care and procedures at home;				
	Home visits.				
A C S	Monthly monitoring of all the families under their responsibility, through home visits;				
	Strengthening the link between individuals/families/community and health services;				
	Mapping your micro-area and registering families;				

Guidance for the community on the right to health and how to access it.				

R = Realise

RP = Partially Realised

NR = Not Realised

Annex IV

CATEGORIES

Staff perception of patient care with the converted model:

The converted model is a combination of the health strategy structure and the health centre, where the ESF starts to work within the CS. There has been a greater bond with the community, a more humanised service and greater access to care. These characteristics provide better quality care for the community and resolve the problems presented. These benefits are common to those found with the ESF in isolation; however, the community agents in particular highlighted the improvement in resolvability, given that they now work within the health centre and take the community's problems directly to the team.

Topics:
...getting to know you better...
...within the community...
...approach...
...trust...
... solve more...
... more humanised...
...easy access...
... ease...
... bond...

Verbalisations:
"I mean, *we* end up getting to know them better because the PSF is about getting to know the **patient, their family, their environment and everything." M.M1**
"the volume of certificates has increased because professionals are getting **sicker in** this new model since they are more involved with their families and their problems, and **the demand for services has increased a lot." AE2**
"Because as a PSF, we get to know the families, we have more dialogue between them, and we know the situation of each one. So when the patient arrives here at the health centre, you already know why, what they're talking about, because of the experience inside their home, because from making home visits so much, we already know, we know the situation of that patient, and at the health centre, when you provide care like this, you don't know the person **who arrives." AXT105**
"One of the positive things about the PSF is the agents, because they're inside the community, they see the situation, the problems in the community and they bring them to us." M.M1
"There was a closer relationship with the community." N.A3
"The trust we gain from the patient." N.Au2
"I think that together with the team we can solve more of the patient's problems today." N.A3

"Resolubility has improved. Now we can give feedback to the population." N.A1
"The positive thing I think *is* that we work with the patient, their family and get to know them well. I like this integration. We don't just provide guidance, we get to know the conditions in which these patients live, so we can adapt to them too. We have a bond with them, a kind of family bond. We make money to help buy filters and food. We do a bazaar, we do everything, cleaning, etc." **Nau4**

66

"I think that together with the team we can solve more of the patient's problems today." Na3
"Another thing is that the preventive part has improved, because that's where we work most with the community." NA3
"When you go into people's homes, you start to see socio-economic issues, cultural issues, family members, which makes it easier for you to provide care and conduct yourself. When you provide care, you know that there are certain guidelines that there's no point in giving because people don't do them. So this makes it much easier" AE1

"The service has become more humanised" A.E2
"The PSF is better, because in the CS we had a lot of difficulty with bedridden patients who couldn't get to the health unit, we had no way of getting to the patient and here it's easier. "AXT102
"They have easier access" N.Au3
"The ease both of getting there and of getting what you want." MEF1 "And the visit is good, because they feel, how do you say, privileged, important when we go there, and we know the environment where they live, right. So it's easier for you to deal with their illnesses, you know, to deal with the situation." MDR1
"The positive points are that the population has more access, you know, to certain programmes, for example, hypertensive patients are monitored, they don't keep changing doctors, each one gives them a different medicine, you know, you don't know, I mean, we end up getting to know them better because the PSF is about getting to know the patient, their family, their environment and everything." MDR1
"It created a greater bond between professionals and the community. When it was just a health centre, the professional didn't have a bond with the patient. Whoever you saw came in, left their complaint and left" AE1
"I believe that patients have found it easier to book appointments, more access and also the issue of patients being able to book appointments and not wait too long." Nau3
"[care] has become more targeted, so only that doctor follows up with that patient, so the doctor knows more about what they're dealing with and the patient doesn't have to start from scratch when they have to see the doctor again, because of their history." Nau3
"Having the vaccine, medication and everything from the health centre helps the PSF a lot, right?" MDR1 "Medication, injections and everything are all here, you know, *the* administrative part, the chance of calling a SAMU, something like that is much easier. So because you're located in a centre, you have all the possibilities. You have the vaccination part. So that's helped a little with the FHP. Because we can solve everything here, we don't need to go anywhere else." MDR1
"Because the number of doctors has increased, (...) because the doctors are general practitioners, they don't just treat you as a doctor, just as a gynaecologist, they treat you as a whole, you know? So it's better for the patient, instead of having to make an appointment with a gynaecologist or a doctor, they just make an appointment and it solves their problem, you know? It was good in that respect." M.Au3:
"It's good here because patients know who their doctor is, who their nurse is, who their team is." M.M1
"There is always one patient or another who tries to make what is simple difficult." A. Au2 "I think the population should value this and they don't, I don't see many difficulties in getting appointments or tests, because I have a health plan, I pay a lot and I get an appointment every two months and here they get appointments overnight, the group didn't even come today (Friday) and the return is for Monday, in the private sector this doesn't exist, you know." MEF1

Team and inter-team work in the general development of functions;

All the health centre's activities, such as the various programmes, work separately according to the team, i.e. each team carries out the health centre's activities for its micro area. The entrance to the health centre is now the team's triage room. Any patient, whether an adult, child or elderly person, must go to the triage room of the team that serves their area of residence. In this room the patient makes an appointment, picks up test results, is referred for care or to hospital depending on their needs.

Some activities are done jointly and there is interaction between the teams whenever one needs help and the other can help, especially in emergencies and technical procedures. So each team has its own decision-making power and planning, but can count on the help of the others in the event of eventualities, and this union provides more flexibility in the service.

There is unity among the staff and teamwork between the various professionals. There are employees who are not part of any team, such as security guards, cleaners, nutritionists, social workers and dentists, who interfere with the good work of the teams. The ACS once again appears as a differential and takes on a more valued role with the conversion.

Topics:
...work as a team...
...separate areas...
...responsible for a micro-area...
...site staff...
...entrance door...
...one team supporting the other...
...there is this exchange...
... valuing the ACS...
...other teams...
...the cleaning ladies...
...the security staff...
... the watchmen...
... I can help...
... teamwork...
...together...
...union...
...companionship...

Verbalisations:

"The biggest change is that here you work as a team. In the traditional system you have a room for **each speciality and in the converted system the team has a room with all the specialities." Nau2 "So the women's programme, the** adult programme, the hypertension programme all **worked** and they still do, but in **separate areas,** in separate blocks with **different PSF** teams." **MAX4**
"Today each team *is* responsible for a micro-area and gets to know the community (...) It's that thing of walking down the street and talking, shaking hands with people, saying hello, saying goodbye. You become their nurse, part of the family, you know? You stop being a stranger, you stop being **"the nurse", the untouchable doctor, and you become that person who starts to** have freedom, and **then you go deeper into the problems, into the cause of those problems." AE1**
"Everything has changed. Before, the patient would come with a complaint, if it was a woman she would be seen in the women's room, a child in the children's room and an adult in the medical clinic. Then there was the adult room. Today it's like this: The family that belongs to that team is seen in a single room. Children, adults, the elderly and teenagers all have the same entrance door. Now the patient is no longer separated by age group, but by where they live. Depending on where they live, they will be seen by the **local team.** It's like that now." **AE2**
"The entrance door is now the triage of each team. So, from suckling to lactating, they'll enter through that door, if they want prevention, to resolve a fever, they'll go to that room and that's very good. And from that room, depending on the need, he'll be booked in, seen or referred to hospital depending on the situation, and he'll be seen by the doctor in the **area." AE1**
"The possibility of decentralising decision-making. I've always argued in favour of decentralising decision making for each team. I think it has to be decentralised because when it comes to managing intra-team resources, you can adapt to the situation experienced by your clients, in your catchment area. I think that's a very good way to go, you know? The possibility of being able to put together strategies (...) That's good, decentralising, because those at the top are the ones who see the problems of the population being **served the** most." **- AM1**

"I do the dressings for our team, and sometimes if the other nurse from the other team isn't free I do the dressings for the **other teams as well." AE1**

"I think that teams have to work not individually, but synergistically and support each other. It's one team supporting another**. Of course, working for their clientele and in the **end working for everyone." - AM1**

"The technician who is currently receiving this patient will check with the other teams to see if there is a** vacancy for another doctor in the emergency department for this patient. **There's this exchange in** relation to emergencies. And in this way, the doctor will attend to any emergencies that arise, whatever the area. **There's** no **division!" AE1**

"We used to be kind of cast aside. With this** conversion we became more involved in the health centre's activities and our work improved a lot. So with the conversion there was a greater **appreciation of the CHAs." NA1**

"This centre is extremely clean, very well looked after, the cleaning girls take great care** of it. Working in a clean environment is something we like **too." AE1**

"The security staff** create a very good bond with the staff and are very **helpful, which is an advantage." AE1**

"The work of the security guards**. They keep patients well informed about the health centre, they **tell patients where to go, they help patients a lot." ATI**

"The staff I can help** orientate the patients within the team post and also about the teams. Because patients don't come here just to see the team, they come to get medicines and other things too. Appointments, vaccinations, pharmacies, dressings, **exam appointments - all this doesn't need the team." ATI**

"Teamwork** [is a positive point], because what we can't resolve we pass on to the group and we interact. Not just with our group, but there's the nutritionist, the social service, the dentist. The role of the CHWs who bring the problems to us, because they're on the streets and know the reality better than we do." **Nau4**

"decisions are always taken together." - AM1**

"Teamwork, because what we can't solve we pass on to the group and **we interact." N.Au2**

"It's *the* unity of the teams that allows us greater flexibility." M.Aul**

"[A positive **point**] is the **unity of the teams" MAX 3**

"It's very good here because all the employees are very united, one is always **helping the other." Mau4**

"Companionship is everything, right, in the teams." MDR1**

"The relationship between civil servants. The work environment for me is very good." - AM1**

Influence of personal motivation and the contribution of professionals to the running of the centre and personal opinions on conversion;

The success of the work often depends on the goodwill of the professional. Despite the difficulties encountered in the network, the motivation and dedication of employees make a difference. Some professionals are resistant to change and show dissatisfaction, while on the other hand there are extremely positive evaluations.

Among the favourable opinions, this new model is seen as more labour-intensive for the employee and, in general, better for the patient. Among the unfavourable, there are those who say that it was better before and that the division into micro-areas leaves part of the population disadvantaged.

Topics:
...goodwill...
...will...
...another peak...
...on behalf of the employees...
...very good...
...for love...
...a bit of a mess...
...difference...

...it would be better...
...that would be great...
...I think it's best...
...terrible...
...resistance...
...they wouldn't accept it...
...lack of interest...
...I fell in love...
...ideal...
...great...
...well...
...more focused...
...excellent service...
...likes it a lot...

Verbalisations:
"Very often the goodwill of the professional doesn't let the patient leave without an answer." ATI
"I think the biggest positive point is *the* **will of** the professionals we have. Because despite all the difficulties, all the wear and tear of the conversion, it wouldn't have happened if the professionals here didn't really want it. (...) the quality of the staff **here. Staff who want to do something, who believe in it and try."** AE1
"So, the question of servers being determined. I think the biggest positive point is the **willingness of** the professionals **we have."** A.E1
"...there are many professionals **here who are committed to what they do. "**AXT103
"You come with all your energy, wanting to do the right thing. The group today is already demotivated. They've had a **different drive. But you keep going 'from strength to strength', and there comes a time when** you stop, there's **nowhere else to go and you pick up again."** AE1
"The staff work well, most of them are calm even though they haven't been **trained** for the **programme."** AA2
"And I've said this several times that this health centre works well because of the staff because with the difficulties, if it were any other type of staff, if it weren't such **dedicated staff, I would have said: 'Oh, you're overloaded and I don't care, I'm not going to do it right', but since the staff here, most of them already** have **a specialisation in** family health, those who don't are doing it, so everyone is very determined, they're very committed, they believe that family health really is good, it has to work and we're **carrying the health centre on our backs."** MEF1
"So, despite all the difficulties, I think this Health Centre is still **very good..."** MEF1
"the people here, they really come to work for love" M.Au4
"Here it's like a prototype of a PSF, right? Because it was supposed to be, it was supposed to work well, but it's just a **bit of a mess."** MEF1
"The difference is just that the teams have been split up." N.A4
"To tell you the truth, I think it was better before." NA4
"In fact, most [of the employees] here would do away with this programme if they could, it would be great for them." M.Au1
"Oh, *the* **way it was before for the employee I think it's better,** but for the patient the PSF way today is better, because for the employee it was easier, for you to deal, to work only with the medical clinic or only with paediatrics, only with pregnant women, now you don't, now you work with everyone, you know, so it's tougher." **MAX4**
"Bad. Because I'm only going to attend to that little group, that little block and the rest **be damned. And patients often complain about that."** MAX 1
"...if it really worked as intended I think it would be very good for both the **servers and the community."** MEF1
"There is still resistance from some. There's resistance to actually converting and changing attitudes. **For**

example, "I'm an old employee, I've been in the secretariat for 20 years and I don't think this is going to work. 'I'm not going to change, I don't want to change'." And that kind of resistance." AA1

"There is still resistance from some employees. They've started training the older staff, so there's been better acceptance, because before they didn't accept it, it was very difficult. Before we only visited, we did everything outside the post." A.A1

"As a negative point I would highlight the lack of interest of some professionals in joining the new system. But I think most of them are already getting on track." NA3

"There is a lack of interest among some professionals in joining the new system." N.A3

"After I saw PSF, I fell in love with it. I think all the health centres in the Federal District should have PSF, because the team is great." Naul

"I think it's the ideal programme, as long as we have professionals and structure." Nau4 "I thought it was great, because it's a health centre that provides excellent care. So much so that people just want to come here." NA2

"If you do some research you'll find people who liked it and those who didn't, but you can't please everyone. But overall I think it was good. I can't say it's excellent because we don't have enough doctors to cater for the whole population." AT2

"I think it's improved, because it's become more focussed. The professionals in that room only see people from that team. It's more organised. It's more focussed, so only that doctor sees that patient." N.Au4

"It's a health centre that provides excellent care." N.A2

"Another positive point is that people accept this programme, they really like it." A.A1

Reflections on the conversion process;

The greatest difficulties encountered arose from the pioneering situation. With no model to follow and no prior training for employees, the conversion process became traumatic. Personal efforts and several attempts led to the creation of what is done today and many employees have already adapted to the new model.

The population also had a period of adjustment; at first they complained a lot. The educational meetings were used to clarify the new way the health centre works and the new division into teams. Some still don't understand why they can't be seen by the doctor if he's there, just because he's not their doctor.

Themes:

...role models...

...training...

...we tried...

...horrible...

...adapt...

...suffering...

...depression...

getting sick...

...conflicts...

...traumatic...

...difficult...

...confused...

...stress...

...tense...

...exhausting...

...labour-intensive...

...something new...

...patient didn't understand...

...people complained...

...neither a centre nor a PSF...

Verbalisations:

"**We didn't have a model to follow**. We had no technical support. We made a lot of mistakes, we had a lot of wear and tear, a lot of conflict. Sometimes it was one way, sometimes it was another. One day we thought: I think **this will work." AE2**

"**What I think got in the way was that the staff weren't** prepared. So much so that they weren't even trained. To this day, some of them find it hard to accept, there are those who say it won't work. There was a lack of **training." AA2**

"**They implemented a system without training us, you** see. So people really got stressed out, I was one who had high blood pressure, I had to take medication because **I tried to do as much as I could and I couldn't." M.Au4**

"**And because we** didn't have any kind of **training**, we were simply told **'Today it's a Health Centre, tomorrow it won't be any more, it's a PSF. So the** conversion **happened overnight.** And another thing is that there was no training, so it became a tumultuous thing, a more difficult thing, not now, now everyone here is more adapted to the **situation, but in the beginning it was horrible. Sad." MAX4**

"**We tried** one way and it didn't work, so we tried another. We tried to organise the medication one way and it didn't work, so we went back and tried another way. I think **this teamwork between all the teams is what made the PSF work." AT2 "Now for the staff it was awful,** [laughs].... Because everything that's new brings frustration and a lot of it. We had no preparation, no support, they just came in and said, do it. And we had to do it the way we could, we tried various ways, until we found a **way that worked. But now it's smooth sailing." MAX4**

"**I thought I wouldn't fit in**. But when I managed to settle in and show my **quality, then it was good."** Naul

"**You have no idea how painful it** was to turn this place into a PSF, it was a war. Until **the technicians understood that it was no longer a health centre, but a PSF, it was a long struggle.** Until the ACSs, who were from Zerbini, understood that they were now from the secretariat and that we were going to **work together, it was a struggle. It was fight after fight. Very exhausting." AE1 "Almost 90 per cent of the professionals went into depression** while taking medication, it's no joke, **they were even dismissed, with a crisis, no one could take the stress." AE1 "The lack of standardisation of services initially led to a lot of conflict." N.Au2 "But the conversion** was very **traumatic for us. A lot of problems." AE2 "It was difficult** for many civil **servants to understand the transformation." NA3**

"**I think it's improved, now, it's improved a lot, in the beginning it was** a bit **confusing,** they didn't know, now they don't, now everyone's adapted, everyone knows, so it's **easier." MAX4**

"**Total stress, [laughs...]" MAX4**

"**Today, now that we've adapted, it's better, we feel a lighter atmosphere, before it was** very tense." MAX4

"**the conversion for the patient I believe was very good, but for the staff** I believe it was **stressful."** MAX4

"**At first it was a bit of a struggle,** people complained and everything. But then we're seeing that it's better. They feel better. I mean, who wouldn't want to know their doctor, their nurse, where to go for help, right? Because **understand what would happen: 'Oh, I'm seen by so-and-so', then I see so-and-so who's off duty, the other one has gone somewhere else and he doesn't know. And** here, we know who I am, we know who the nurse is, we know who the **community workers are." MDR1**

"**And for** *the* community it was **something new. When the community arrived and we said 'you don't have to come here anymore, you have to come somewhere else', I spent about three months using half of the** educational meetings to explain what was going on, the new way the **health centre worked, to try and ease the stress." AE1**

"**And sometimes the patient doesn't understand** much because sometimes there's a doctor from the other team and the one from your team isn't there, so they don't understand why they won't be seen even though there is a **doctor." AT2**

"**At first it was a** bit of a chore, **people complained about everything." M.M1**

"**We're neither a centre nor a PSF.** Because I worked for many years as a family doctor in a little post office that used to be a PSF. So for me, this isn't a PSF. But it's not a centre either, so...?" MDR1

The relationship between physical structure, staff and demand on the quality of care;

Some staff point to the increase in the number of employees with the conversion, but there has been an expansion of the area without increasing the number of teams and there is a greater demand than the capacity of the teams. The health centre itself doesn't have enough physical structure for the teams, they have to share some rooms, and this and the growing demand is reflected in the delay in care, the prioritisation of risk groups and hinders promotion and prevention actions.

Demand also helps to shape the service, since patients prioritise medical consultations and don't have a culture of health promotion and prevention.

Topics:
...new area...
...every demand...
...complaint...
...patient mentality...
...only gets a consultation...
...a lot of people...
...physical space...
...structure...
...professional...
...support...
...audiovisual...
...medicines...

Verbalisations:
"It's not a 100 per cent area. There's a new settlement **area** that doesn't have its own teams, these areas ended up being distributed among the teams that already exist. So today the population of out-of-area patients and patients in the team's area is almost the same. So the team that had to cater for a certain population is catering for **twice as many." AE2**
"We'd have to have a team for rural areas, which we don't have. If there was coverage of these areas it would be better because we would end up joining too. In addition to our micro-areas, I end up seeing patients from the settlements and rural areas. So there's an overload that **jeopardises care in my area of responsibility." AE1**
"Here there are teams 7, 9 and 10, there are only three teams to meet all the demand, it's impossible. That's the biggest difficulty here. This generates a lot of **complaints from patients** who want to be attended to for **all their needs." Naul**
"And this issue of not having a team trained to attend to the 800 and 1000. After the settlement there, there was a big increase in **attendance here."MAX3 "The reinforcement of the** local **teams,** the sending of new doctors, the composition of new teams **so that we can run the boat more smoothly." A.M1**

"There are cases of patients who move but continue to use the same address to continue being seen here. There's also the case of relatives of patients from the centre who come to **spend their holidays and (...) use the card as if they were from here." Naul**
"Because the centre is so good, people come from other places to want to be seen here." NA1
"the number of inhabitants served is greater than the health centre's capacity, which compromises the service and generates **complaints among the team" N.Aul**
"Although, as I said, they (patients) complain a lot, saying they can't get an **appointment" A.E1**
"When they start booking, the diary is already full. The patient never gets an appointment, for **example: day I° opens up, on day 3 it's already over." AA2**
"Although, as I said, they (patients) complain a lot, saying they can't get an **appointment" A.E1**
"Sometimes I prefer to work in hospital, because there the patient is sick and needs you, not here the **patient is** mostly healthy and he's rude, uneducated and **wants things on the spot." Naul**
"So the patient always demands the doctor's presence, because they are not yet aware **that health is not**

just about the doctor (...) because they have a view that the doctor is everything." Nau3 "It's still necessary to change the mentality of the assisted patient, who believes more in curative medicine than preventive medicine, which is what the PSF is all about." Nau3

"the aim here is consultation, consultation, consultation, consultation, you don't see this part [promotion and prevention] so we end up not having that. So that's what I miss." MDR1 "Another positive point is the coverage of risk groups (diabetics, hypertensive patients and children), hypertensive patients, for example, 80% coverage, only we don't say 100% because some work a lot and sometimes can't take part." A.AI:
"You can only get an appointment if you're hypertensive, diabetic, pregnant or a child up to 2 years old. After 2 years, you can't." AA2
Nau2: Here we don't have the structure to cater for young drug addicts, nor where to send them for treatment.
"And so the negative point is this problem that we have too many people to attend to in the Health Centre and it takes away from the main focus which is basic care, which is part of promotion and education."MAX3
"There are many times when we can't leave here because there's only one doctor, we can't go out for a visit." MDR1
"... in the PSF there's the prenatal care programme, the CD programme, the group programme, you know, group meetings, pregnant women's meetings, CD meetings, visits, you know, and here we don't have as many opportunities for that." MDR1
"The centre is small for the high demand." N.A2:
"There needs to be a room just for us CHWs." NA2
"The physical space is very small. I think it's too small for three teams." M.M1
"The medication and dressing room is separate from the team, ideally the team should have direct access to these services." Nau2
"If you have to see a patient and give them medication or a vaccine, we don't have rooms for these procedures. These services are concentrated in a single room," Nau4
"The physical space is small. There needs to be a room just for us CHWs." NA2:
"The physical space doesn't help" MDR1
"If more teams come, we won't be able to fit them in. The physical structure can't take it anymore." MEF1

"...I think a maximum of two teams here would be marvellous. It's because of the structure, if it was bigger, it would be 3, but it still wouldn't be able to cope with the demand here." MDR1
"The centre was very cramped with three teams in one place. I don't think it's bad, but it could be better. The fact that three teams are close together doesn't interfere, it's not a problem. The problem is the physical area, which is bad, that makes it difficult." AE1
"But the structure also leaves something to be desired, because the parts are not integrated. The medication and dressing room is separate from the team. Ideally, the team should have direct access to these services." N.Au3
"It needs a proper structure. More rooms. For me, as a member of team 10, if I have to see a patient and give them medication or a vaccine, we don't have rooms for these procedures. These services are concentrated in a single room, because we have no way of dividing them up." N.Au2
"Although we realise that there's always a complaint, because sometimes there's no doctor because he's on sick leave or he's doing a course." Nau3
"What's changed is that now there are more doctors and more nurses." N.A2
"...there are doctors, there are nurses, there are community workers, it's... even though they are overloaded, the team is complete so far." MEF1
"There aren't enough professionals to cater for everyone." A.E2
"There's always a shortage of professionals, especially in medicine." M.Aul "We are faced with various difficulties, various social and economic problems that we can't solve. We've had a social worker

for four months now, and as well as being **a nurse for all these people, you also have to be a psychologist and a social worker** - it's extremely difficult, isn't it? You even get ill. You end up getting ill from the overload." **AE1**

"For example, I have an area that had 4 CHWs and one was moved to GAPESF in the hospital. This left an **uncovered area, I** mean, an area that needed 6, only had 4 and I **lost 1 in the team. That makes it difficult." AE1**

"I believe that the support is still very poor, it has to improve a lot so that we can **really have a PSF (social worker, nutritionist, etc.)." A.E1**

"Sometimes there's nobody in our team." A.A2

"The drinking fountains are missing too." N.A1

"Another point is that there is sometimes a lack of material to work with." A.AI

"There's very little **material.** Because even what we have going on, medication that used to be in short supply, is now in short supply why? Because demand has increased, the number of people has increased, but the number of people coming to the centre hasn't increased. And apart from equipment, **blood pressure monitors, blood glucose monitors and everything else that when it breaks, it goes and doesn't come back, right?" MDR1 "The CHWs who don't have any kind of material don**'t get sunscreen, caps, raincoats, pencils, pens, pads, none of that. They have to work with their **own** resources **and so do we. We work with a lot of things we bring." AE1**

"Oh, for example, we've just given a lecture, there's no audiovisual, there's nothing, there's a blackboard here, but there's no chalk, there's a video there, but there's no tape to play. **So we're just stuck at the bottleneck" MEF1**

"And the working conditions, lack of material, lack of pens and erasers, that comes once a **year. There's a lack of bags and uniforms, which we make ourselves, because they don't come." AGT10**

"There's always **medication** here, thank God. It's always been **very** difficult for **these things to come here. M.Au4**

"We need to improve the distribution of medicines, which is sometimes lacking." A.E1: **"The pharmacy, which lacks a lot of medication, the delay in taking tests." M.A1:**

Continuing education;

There is currently no continuing education at the health centre. There are occasional initiatives by each team that try to address relevant issues and adhere to the programmes offered by the health department.

Topics:
...training...
...continuing education...

Verbalisations:
"At the centre, training *in* general isn't happening, it's happening in isolation, where each nurse guides their group of CHWs." AE1

"There's no set schedule or frequency. They're actually meetings, even one-off meetings where we talk about a few things, but it doesn't really come down to an educational theme of running a class or doing further training. That's up to the health department itself. But there is an intention on the part of the team to carry out continuing education. We want to prepare these professionals in emergency care so that they can facilitate the care provided by doctors and nurses. What education there is for professionals is provided by the health department itself in specific programmes and when there are events for CHAs to improve and educate them and workshops for doctors, nurses and nursing technicians." - AM1

Influence of existing standardisation and management on strategy performance.

The final potential of this strategy also depends on government investment, the work of other hierarchical levels and the support of regulatory bodies. Productivity assessment is basically quantitative and there is a requirement to see 20 patients per shift, which sometimes restricts the doctor to the consulting room.

The constant changing of the health centre's management leads to discontinuous work and can generate a degree of anxiety in the staff.

The data from the situation room could be better used if it were decentralised and easy to retrieve. The time that the health professional spends on these statistics could be used for health care and there could be an administrative professional trained for this purpose.

Topics:
...invest...
...quality...
...quantity...
...it depends...
...director...
...restricts...
...required...
...management...
...decentralisation...

Verbalisations:
M.Au4: "Whoever manages it, because the regional centre should invest more, you know? Because they know it's something that, in the future, the whole of Brazil will have, right? So it's something that

has been established here. If it's established here, it has to continue here for things to move on in other **places. This should be the first place, the model."**
"Now, a negative point, (...) there are the numbers that 'the people up there are demanding'. And the PSF isn't about numbers, it's about **quality of care." M.M1**
"Because it doesn't just depend on the person who's here, it depends **on** the hospital, it depends on the **routine, delivering and bringing in material" MAX1**
"There should be at least one meeting between the director of GAPESF and all the PSF **coordinators,** and there isn't, there isn't! There's a general meeting at least once a month, so that they are aware of our difficulties. So there are lots of difficulties, and this **demotivates us." AE 1**
"We have to work with the team as public servants to provide the statistics that the department requires of you, which are eminently **quantitative** statistics." - AM1 **"It's often difficult to carry out preventive work because the professional is restricted to the consulting room." ATI**
"There is also a demand that is required by the health department from the professionals, which **is 20 patients per period." - AM1**
"Quantity is not a good service in our area of health. What's important to us is the **quality of the service, of the care." MAX1 "It's because they say 20, it's because** 15 minutes per patient. That's 20 in five hours of service, you know? So the PSF doesn't work like that. It's not about time, it's not about quantity, it's about **quality, the reason, the follow-up." MDR1**
"Certainly, quality is affected, for example, how are you going to be able to talk, get **the patient to open up and everything in a 15-minute consultation?" MDR1**
"It's become fashionable here now to change **heads** every day because of politics. And so someone starts a job, lays the foundations, things go along, and the next thing you know, tomorrow it's no more, someone else comes in, with different ideas, and everything starts all over again, you know? And we have to end up adapting to the way of working, so this leads to frustration and indignation, and there end up being **disagreements between employees." M.Au3**
"The boss doesn't stop **here, so something starts and doesn't finish." AGT10**
"The constant change of director is also bad, because when you adapt you **change. A stone that rolls a lot doesn't create slime." NA3**
"There would have to be a situation room not just for the centre but for each team. I think the process of

decentralisation enhances action through information and then allows you to recentralise it. So if you have decentralisation in your situation room, you know the profile of your area, you know the profile of the other team's area and the manager can put this together. So I don't think it would have to be a single room for the centre, it would have to be a room for each team. (...) I don't think this kind of service should be delegated to a health professional, but to an administrative professional. The health professional whose knowledge could be used for something else, such as care and more meetings, for example. But the part of simply retrieving information that the system should give us is already done and doesn't cause these problems in the system. This would be a **huge** improvement for us." - **AM1**

Computerisation

There was an overlap of changes. During the conversion, CSSam 03 underwent a computerisation process, again without adequate training and with a lot of conflict, the system is slow, goes offline frequently, does not have adequate technical support, but it is contributing to better assistance.

Topics:
...computerisation...
...computer...
...electronic...

Verbalisations:
"Computerisation **in health is excellent."** **A.M1**
"I had a hard time at first because I didn't know how to use a computer, because I thought I **would never need one." Naul**
"Then came computerisation, which meant moving from paper to electronic media. The system is good, but it's very slow. Extremely slow. It crashes a lot. Then the professional has to go out and say that the system is down and the population doesn't realise that the problem is with the **information and blames the service staff for the delay." AE2**
"I think computerisation has been important, because now we have access to tests much faster, to the results. Access to patient records has also improved with computerisation, a lot of tests used to disappear, records used to disappear and now with **computerisation there's none of that." MAX4**
"Patients who have their prenatal care here at the clinic, fill in the card and do everything here, **when she's going to have a baby in hospital they already know who she had her prenatal care with,** the tests that were ordered, you **know,** that's the advantage of the **electronic** medical record.**" AE2 "Another thing I like about this computer** is its practicality, because it's very difficult to **handle paperwork." Naul**
"There are flaws in the system regarding the computerisation of the health centre, because it was just thrown at us and the system simply has no support. It takes a long time for us to do the triage and the patients don't understand that it's not our fault and it's the system's fault. Sometimes the patient stays in the room for more than 15 minutes before we can get them booked in." **Nau3**
"It's very difficult to progress on the computer, you spend a lot of time. This programme is very slow, even for me who doesn't know much about it. It had to be a faster programme. Another thing is that it gives off too much air, you're attending and suddenly everything goes down, so you have to stop attending the patient until they come back. If it had a **more efficient** monitoring centre, **maybe that would solve the problem." Naul**
"So, in terms of the computer, if there was someone to give support on the computer, the **best service was the computer." M.Au4**

Annex V

Participant Observation

Doctors

Team	7	9	10
Knowledge of the Referral Against Referral System	REALISE	REALISE	REALISE
Execution of basic health and epidemiological surveillance actions	REALISE	REALISE	REALISE
Consultation, diagnosis and treatment of individuals and families	REALISE	REALISE	REALISE
Filling in the activity production log	REALISE	REALISE	REALISE
Home visits	PARTIALLY REALISED	PARTIALLY REALISED	PARTIALLY REALISED
Participation in the training, capacity building and continuing education process for the teams	PARTIALLY REALISED	PARTIALLY REALISED	PARTIALLY REALISED
Planning educational activities	REALISE	REALISE	REALISE

Nurses

Team	7	9	10
Monitoring of registration and updating of data by CHAs	PARTIALLY REALISED	PARTIALLY REALISED	REALISES PARTIALLY
Helping to organise the basic health unit	REALISES	REALISES	REALISES
Carrying out basic health and epidemiological surveillance actions	PARTIALLY REALISED	PARTIALLY REALISED	REALISES PARTIALLY
Planning, execution, coordination	REALISES	REALISES	REALISES
Monitoring and evaluation of nursing care actions for individuals and their families	REALISES	REALISES	REALISES
Promoting training and continuing education for the nursing team	PARTIALLY REALISED	PARTIALLY REALISED	REALISES PARTIALLY
Home visits	PARTIALLY REALISED	PARTIALLY REALISED	PARTIALLY REALISED

Nursing Technicians

Team	7	9	10
Identifying families at risk and monitoring their individuals together with the ACS	NOT REALISED	NOT REALISED	NOT REALISED
Cleaning, disinfection, sterilisation, conservation and storage of the service's material and equipment	PARTIALLY REALISED	PARTIALLY REALISED	PARTIALLY REALISED
Nursing care and procedures at home	REALISE	REALISE	REALISE
Home visits	PARTIALLY REALISED	PARTIALLY REALISED	PARTIALLY REALISED

Community Health Agents

Team	7	9	10
Monthly monitoring of all the families under their responsibility, through home visits	PARTIALLY REALISED	PARTIALLY REALISED	REALISES PARTIALLY
Strengthening the link between individuals/families/community and health services	REALISES	REALISES	REALISES
Mapping your micro-area and registering families	REALISES	REALISES	REALISES
Guidance for the community on the right to health and how to access it	PARTIALLY REALISED	PARTIALLY REALISED	PARTIALLY REALISED

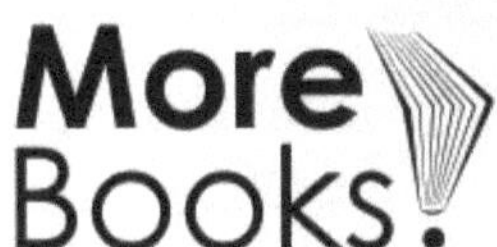

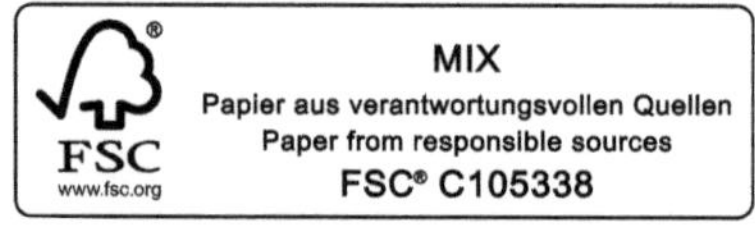

Printed by Books on Demand GmbH, Norderstedt / Germany